SKILLS FOR CARE PLANNING

Also in the *Education for Care* series:

EDUCATION FOR CARE

SKILLS FOR CARE PLANNING
Teaching the Skills of the Nursing Process

DIANE J MARKS-MARAN BSc SRN DipN(Lond) RNT
Senior Tutor, Curriculum Development and Research
St Bartholomew's School of Nursing
London

With contributions by
SYLVIA P DOCKING MA SRN SCM RNT
Principal, Riverside College of Nursing, London
Honorary Lecturer, King's College London (KQC)

TERRY MAUNDER BA RMN RNT
Tutor, St Bartholomew's School of Nursing, London

JANICE SCOTT SRN DipN(PartA) RCNT RNT
Tutor, Charing Cross School of Nursing, London

SCUTARI PRESS
London

© Scutari Press 1988

A division of Scutari Projects Ltd, the publishing company of the Royal College of Nursing

First published 1988

British Library Cataloguing in Publication Data

Marks-Maran, Diane J.
Skills for care planning: teaching the skills of the nursing process.
(Education for care series).
1. Interpersonal relationships.
Communication–For nursing
I. Title   II. Series
302.2′024613

ISBN 1 871364 12 4

Typeset by Woodfield Graphics, Arundel, West Sussex
Printed and bound by Biddles Ltd., Guildford

Table of Contents

Preface

Care planning within the framework of the nursing
process has developed remarkably in the last decade.
What does it take to plan and give care in this way?
Undoubtedly, it takes a good deal of knowledge—about
illness, human biology, the psychological response to
illness, sociology, pathology, and so forth. There is little
doubt that it also takes skill—skill in carrying out
procedures safely, skill at relating to people in distress,
skill in managing staff, and various other skills.

This book is an attempt to address what is sometimes
called the 'people skills' required to plan and give care—
skills such as those about relating to others, coping with
stress and being aware of one's responses and feelings—
rather than the knowledge base or practical tasks of nursing or of care planning.

All nurses, whether they are clinical nurses, managers
or teachers, have a role in helping others to develop and
learn. There are many personal and interpersonal skills
involved in care planning and in giving care in a
sensitive, individualised way. Unfortunately, many nurse
teachers have little help or guidance in how to develop
these skills either in themselves or in others. The same is
true for nurse managers and clinical nurses who are
trying to help their staff to develop. The aim of this book,
therefore, is to identify the changing role of those who

teach others, to identify the 'people skills' involved in care planning and to offer practical suggestions on how to help others to develop these skills so that care planning can be carried out in a more humanistic way.

The book is divided into four sections. In Section I (Chapters 1–4), Chapter 1 explores the relationship between care planning and nursing education. Chapter 2 examines changing teaching methods and changing ideas on what teaching and learning are about. Experiential teaching methods are introduced in Chapter 3, and Chapter 4 offers a model for teaching interpersonal skills.

Section II contains Chapters 5–7. Each examines a particular stage in the nursing process and identifies the personal and interpersonal skills required to assess patients, to make nursing diagnoses and plan and evaluate care. Section III (Chapters 8–10) looks at areas of personal growth and development required of nurses so that they may know themselves better in order to relate to others more effectively. The three areas examined in this section are: ethical decision-making (Chapter 8), self-awareness (Chapter 9), and basic life skills (Chapter 10).

Section 4 (Chapters 11 and 12) has been contributed by teachers who describe examples of teaching programmes designed to help others to develop the personal and interpersonal skills required for care planning and humanistic nursing. In Chapter 11, Terry Maunder and Janice Scottt explore a skills workshop for introductory course nurses in basic nursing. Chapter 12, written by Sylvia Docking, examines a nursing process skills workshop for nursing officers using the approaches suggested in the earlier part of the book.

An appendix on role play and a detailed reading and resource list for anyone wishing to develop further techniques in teaching care planning skills complete the book.

This book is intended as a helpful companion volume to *Nursing Care Plans: The Nursing Process at Work* by Jenny Hunt and Diane Marks-Maran. Whereas *Nursing Care*

Plans serves as a practical guide for implementing care planning, *Skills for Care Planning* is for those involved in teaching the 'people skills' of care planning, whether this teaching is being undertaken in a classroom or in the clinical area. It offers exercises to help people to know themselves better, manage stress, develop strategies to act as an advocate of the patient, feel confident, celebrate strengths, trust themselves and others and feel good about themselves. By developing all these attributes, a nurse will be in a stronger position to give the type of humanistic, individualised care towards which we all strive.

As nursing travels into the 21st century, one can only hope that those who teach nurses will realise that the key to teaching nursing at any level or in any location is to enable nurses to develop their personal skills. The type of teaching put forward in this book should be a major part of nursing and nursing education.

For this is what the nursing process is all about.

Diane J. Marks-Maran
1988

Acknowledgements

This book has been lurking in my brain, heart and soul for many years, starting with the time I began to realise that individualised care planning is not just an intellectual task, that is, an end product to be written on pieces of paper, but is also a personal ethos—a statement of the values we hold about individual rights, sharing control with patients and the need for nurses to be able to relate to patients on a person-to-person level rather than a nurse-to-patient level. If you, the reader, open this book expecting it to tell you how to write a care plan, you may find yourself none the wiser by the time you reach the end of it. Instead, it is for all of you who wish to explore your own personal skills, self-awareness and the way you relate to others so that you may identify the human skills you might wish to develop to enable you to care for others as individuals and to relate to others on a person-to-person level. It is a book about helping people to know themselves and others better rather than how to carry out any tasks of nursing.

The very fact that I have been able to write this book I owe to many people who have played such a large part in my own personal development, especially Sylvia Docking, Liz Keighley, Brigid Breckman, Janice Scott, Terry Maunder, Meg Bond, Juliette and the group, Judith Sunderland, Sue MacWhirter and Anne Currell. Within these pages are their support and love.

D M-M

Section I

Chapter 1

Care Planning and Nurse Education

Nurse education is concerned with teaching and learning at both basic and postbasic level and as such plays an important part in the implementation of a care planning system. In the second edition of their book *Nursing Care Plans: the Nursing Process at Work*, Hunt & Marks-Maran (1986) devote a chapter to the role of nurse education in care planning. Many of the ideas and arguments presented in that chapter emphasise that nurse educators do indeed have a large role to play in enabling nurses to plan nursing care in a way which is individual to each patient and which systematically identifies and acts upon people's needs.

Teaching care planning: who, what, when and how?

Who teaches care planning? One of the most important concepts in teaching care planning skills is that the teacher is wherever the learner is. In the case of care planning, nurse teachers, clinical nurses and nurse managers all have a part to play in enabling students (basic and postbasic) to develop care planning skills. This teaching can take place in a formal classroom setting (see Chapter 11) or at the bedside. It happens in many ways—by the student observing skills being put into practice by others, by the student experiencing the use of a particular skill and reflecting upon how she feels that skill is developing, by discussion and by a variety of other learning methods. This highlights the need for all those who are involved with students to be skilled themselves in care planning in order to be effective role models for those who are learning. It also highlights the need for teaching to take place in a wide variety of settings and using a wide variety of teaching methods.

This book is based on several assumptions made by the author about care planning. These are that:

- Nurse teachers, nurse managers and clinical nurses all believe that individualised, systematic care planning is a desirable thing.
- Nurse managers and clinical nurses believe that they have an important teaching role in helping others to develop care planning skills.
- Teaching care planning skills can take place in the relative safety of the classroom, using appropriate teaching methods, as well as at the bedside.

All those involved with nurses or patients become teachers of care planning skills whether it is through their own practice or through deliberate teaching strategies. Each clinical nurse, manager or teacher provides a different dimension to enable care planning skills to be developed in others. Practising nurses should have the opportunity and, indeed, the desire to develop further their own care planning skills either through direct experience or through structured teaching programmes. Nurse teachers should do the same by keeping themselves up to date and by experiencing new and different teaching methods which are appropriate to helping others to develop care planning skills.

What are care planning skills? When the nursing process was first described as an individualised, systematic way of thinking about and organising nursing care, an attempt was made to incorporate this new concept into clinical practice and nurse education. Some hospitals and health districts responded by organising structured educational programmes to enable all staff to learn about this new approach to nursing. Many, however, did not, thinking that whatever skills were required to practise nursing in this way could be 'picked up' with time and experience. Indeed, many skills can be learnt in this way. Most schools of nursing incorporated something about the nursing process into their programmes, especially since the National Boards (formerly the General Nursing Council) require it. This input, however, was largely related to didactic teaching sessions about theory, such as identification and explanation of the stages of the nursing process. In short, the nursing process became another task because it was taught like a task. This is best seen, perhaps, in many of the ways in which care plans were incorporated into basic nursing programmes. Nurses' performance and progress were assessed by the use of improved, written care plans, teaching sessions were organised on how to fill in the forms, and so on. Little attempt has been made to relate this process of nursing with the processes required to carry it out. The nursing process is a dynamic activity, not a set of forms to be filled in, which is jointly engaged in by nurses and patients and which requires a wide range of sophisticated skills which nurses continually need to develop if their practice is to be patient centred. Little attempt has been made in the past to dissect the nursing process into its component skills and to identify ways of enabling nurses to develop these skills. Taking a nursing history or writing a care plan is a task—but to do it well, and in a way which allows a patient to grow and progress towards maximum health and independence, requires certain skills. It is the systematic development of these skills which appears to be missing from nursing education.

Because of this, there appears to be almost a tacit belief that whatever skills are required to assess patients, identify nursing problems, make nursing diagnoses, implement and evaluate care, already exist within all nurses and all that is needed is factual information about the patient and the stages of the nursing process. But experience tells us, some ten years on, that our understanding of the nursing process and care planning has developed tremendously and our insight into the knowledge and skills required to practise nursing in this way has also grown. Each stage of the nursing process requires its own enormous range of sophisticated skills if one is to be able to give the kind of individualised nursing care which patients deserve. Nurses need a wide range of skills and must have the opportunity to discover where their strengths and weaknesses lie with respect to these skills and how they can go about the business of developing those which they wish to improve. The implication for teaching programmes is tremendous because each nurse (trained or untrained) will be at a different level of development for various skills at any given time. New teaching methods must be used which allow for these differences.

Teaching care planning is more than just explaining the various stages of the nursing process, and is also more than just teaching the tasks (such as taking a nursing history). Instead, it is about providing structured learning opportunities in a wide variety of settings which will enable each nurse to develop all the skills which are inherent in the nursing process.

Some of the skills required to assess patients, make nursing diagnoses, plan and evaluate care are as follows:

- Observation
- Interviewing
- Priority-setting
- Problem-solving
- Interpersonal skills, e.g.

     listening
     asking appropriate questions
     confronting
     encouraging self-discovery
     information-giving
     supporting
     giving advice
- Goal-setting
- Evaluating
- Assertiveness
- Decision-making
     managerial
     ethical
- Negotiating
- Self-awareness
- Self-assessment

This list is by no means exhaustive but each of the skills listed has to be developed by a nurse if she is to become an effective and sensitive care planner and care giver. Specific time and learning experiences, and in a higher proportion than exists at present, must be given throughout training and throughout a nurse's career. None of the skills identified in the above list is more important than any other—all must be developed equally, and very specific teaching methods must be employed in order that they can be learnt.

When and where should care planning skills be taught and learnt? The care planning skills identified in the previous section do not have an identifiable end point. There is no stage at which any nurse can say 'I've reached the point where I have fully developed my problem-solving (or listening or interviewing) skills.' Each new care planning situation will require a unique approach by the nurse as she listens and interacts, because each new patient is unique. Thus, the development of the various skills should start at the beginning of training and allow the nurse to identify the stage already reached with regard to each skill. This development must keep pace with each individual throughout training and her career. Development in one skill area may occur more quickly or more slowly than development in another. So long as there are people requiring preventive, curative, rehabilitative or continuing nursing care, continued development of all care planning skills is required.

Care planning and the nursing process are often poorly understood because they have become tasks in themselves and have not succeeded in coming up to expectations. Nurses are being expected to practise nursing in this systematic way without being given the opportunity either to identify the skills required to do so or to develop these skills. Essentially, the end product (such as the completion of a nursing history form or writing a problem-solving essay) has become the high priority, regardless of the quality of the information obtained from the history and the use made of it.

To change the situation to one which actively seeks to help people to develop these very specific skills throughout their training and career, teachers, managers and clinical nurses can do several things. Firstly, skills development of this nature must be given priority by curriculum planners and by the statutory bodies and time allowed for this in all nursing education programmes. Secondly, nurse managers and clinical nurses must seek to develop their own care planning skills and provide teaching time on wards and units, whenever possible, to allow care planning skills development to take place in a structured way at the bedside. Thirdly, nurse teachers must learn and develop new and more appropriate teaching methods to enable them to help their students develop care planning skills both in the classroom and at the bedside.

The remainder of the book will provide ideas, suggestions and advice on how these three things can be achieved, including a wide range of short, effective teaching activities specifically for use in classroom and bedside teaching.

How can care planning skills be taught? This question is directly related to the development of new and more appropriate teaching methods, suggestions for which make up a large part of the second and third sections of this book. One feature of the shift which is required in teaching methods is introduced here and expanded in Chapter 3.

Historically, the intention of nursing education was to impart information and to ensure development of certain essential psychomotor skills (e.g. doing a dressing). The teaching methods required for these two things are the didactic, lecture-style method and rote learning by demonstration ('Watch me do this and then I'll watch you try to do it exactly the way I did it.').

The nursing process demanded that nurses rethink what nursing means and in order to implement this individualised, total patient care planning system, other skills are required in addition to knowledge and psycho-motor skills. These are the sophisticated care planning skills identified earlier and these do not fit the didactic or demonstration teaching methods. As new skills are incorporated into nursing care and teaching program-mes, we also have to incorporate more appropriate teaching methods to go with these. It is essential to say at the outset that care planning skills and the teaching methods required for their development are intended to enhance, not to replace, traditional teaching methods.

How care planning skills are taught is probably as important as the skills themselves and is quite different from teaching factual information or psychomotor skills. The outcome of a lecture on a particular subject or the demonstration of a psychomotor skill generally has a measurable end; for example, that the student can repeat back the factual information imparted in the lec-ture or demonstrate that she can do the dressing safely and efficiently. Care planning skills do not have these predetermined, identifiable measurable end results. Each nurse can identify where she is in terms of her own development of a particular care planning skill and only she can determine and measure her progress and growth. With a lecture or demonstration the teacher assumes that everyone will come out at the end with the same knowledge and skill. With care planning skills, if appropriate teaching methods are used each nurse will progress at a different rate and will be at different stages of development at the end of each session. Rather than the end product of a predictable outcome, care planning skills are concerned with the process of development, and this process is personal and individual to each nurse. Because of this, the product-centred teaching method, such as the lecture or rote-style demonstration, is inappropriate for teaching care planning skills which are process-centred. Thus, all those who teach care planning skills must themselves learn process-centred teaching methods and their appropriate use.

This has implications for both classroom and ward or bedside teaching. Many nurse teachers and clinical nurses have, themselves, never been taught care planning skills, nor may teachers have had experience of process-centred teaching methods in their teaching training programmes. Both may feel unskilled and uncomfortable either in giving care in this new way or in teaching the skills of care planning. This will be elaborated on in Chapter 2.

Clinical nurses as teachers of care planning skills

Student nurses are notorious for thinking that no one has taught them anything while on a ward because there have been no formal teaching sessions at which a clinical teacher, sister or staff nurse has sat them down and talked at them about a particular disease or subject. Equally, many nurses have been known to say 'I don't have time to do any teaching' when they really mean that they may not have the time or the skill to sit with a group of students and talk to them for half an hour (Thompson & Bridge 1981).

Yet teaching the care planning skills required for systematic, individualised nursing does not necessarily require this formal, sit-in-a-circle approach to ward teaching. Historically, teaching at the bedside has involved reviewing factual information about a disease or treatment, or teaching a particular psychomotor skill—in other words, product-centred teaching sessions. Care planning skills (process-centred), where the development of the skill is a continuing personal process, requires different types of ward-based learning activities which can be organised by trained staff or ward-based teachers.

Qualified nurses can provide these types of activity on the ward in addition to the factual or psychomotor teaching which takes place. The simplest, and perhaps the most effective, way of teaching care planning skills is for a trained nurse to take a student with her whenever she undertakes a care planning activity with a patient. This role model approach is a powerful learning tool. The student can observe this trained nurse, for example, as she interviews a patient on admission. The important part of this learning process for the student, however, is that time is spent after the interview discussing the types of questions used, why the trained nurse phrased questions in a certain way, and so forth. This should be followed up as soon as possible by the student interviewing a patient on admission while the trained nurse watches, after which, the student can discuss her own performance with the trained nurse and plan ways of improving specific parts of her interviewing technique. This is the most essential part of the role model method of teaching: having the opportunity to discuss, try out the skill under supervision, discuss again and plan for future learning. This same process can be used for developing problem-solving, decision-making and most of the other care planning skills. Sharing experiences in this way with a skilled care planner will enable the student to discover her own strengths and weaknesses and find alternative ways of managing care planning situations. One final word of caution: problems will arise if the role model is herself unskilled, for the learner will then observe the wrong type of practice.

Time set aside for formal teaching need not be used only for knowledge- or subject-based teaching but can also be spent on care planning skills development. This can be carried out with any number of students. Many of the exercises and activities in Sections II and III of this book can easily be used in ward teaching sessions for care planning skills development.

Summary

All those involved in teaching nursing have an enormous role to play in care planning. The wide range of sophisticated skills required to plan nursing care in a systematic, individualised way is identified in this chapter, as is the equal role and responsibility that nurse teachers, managers and clinical nurses each have in helping nurses to develop these skills. The skills can be taught in the classroom or at the bedside but require an approach to teaching methods that is different from that used in traditional ward-based teaching.

References

Hunt J M & Marks-Maran D (1986) *Nursing Care Plans: The Nursing Process at Work*. Chichester: John Wiley & Sons

Thompson B & Bridge W (1981) *Teaching Patient Care: A Handbook for the Practising Nurse*. Chichester: John Wiley & Sons

Chapter 2

The Changing Forms of Teaching

Care planning has, as already mentioned, until recently been taught in the classroom in a didactic way. Using a lecture format, teachers have attempted to teach students how to plan nursing care by identifying and describing the stages of the nursing process, leaving the practicalities of care planning for students to 'pick up' on the wards as they went along. Practical teaching has involved showing them how to fill in the forms rather than consciously identifying and developing the skills of care planning.

Imagine the nursing process with no pieces of paper at all—no history forms and no care plans—and imagine also how one might teach the students what it means to assess, make nursing diagnoses, plan and evaluate care in a systematic individualised way when there are no pieces of paper and no documentation on which to focus.

How can one explain nursing assessment to new nurses without a sheet of paper for guidance? Can students develop these assessment skills in other ways without 'being told' or 'shown' them? What other options are there for teaching assessment skills?

In addition, what can be done to help students to develop the ability to identify problems in patients, set priorities and choose appropriate action from a long list of possible alternatives. Remember, all documentation has been thrown away.

What about making decisions? How may students develop the processes involved in decision-making? How may they live comfortably with the decisions they make day by day?

The first step in sorting out these questions is to agree that they highlight the enormous range of skills required to plan effective nursing care. The second step is to acknowledge that present approaches to teaching these skills are inappropriate and that one must be able, so-to-speak, to throw off the shackles of some of our traditional teaching methods in both the classroom and at the bedside, creatively explore other possibilities and in doing so embark upon an exciting journey into new realms of personal and professional skills development.

Alternative teaching strategies

Whether one is a nurse teacher, manager or clinical nurse, one will have a teaching responsibility related to care planning. The premise is, however, that no matter where a nurse is in her career, she has areas of skill development which could be improved or enhanced. Other ways of teaching care planning skills can be explored. Even with thirty or forty students and having only a large classroom to work in it is possible to use this situation creatively and develop process-centred teaching strategies to enable those students to build care planning skills. Equally, these alternative teaching methods need not be confined to the school of nursing nor to nurse teachers. They can be used creatively in the ward situation by clinical teachers, managers or clinical nurses to teach care planning skills to a small group of students.

The fundamental principle behind alternative teaching strategies is that direct, personal experience in trying out a skill will enable the student to feel what it is like, build up confidence in using the skill, identify strengths and weaknesses and to decide for herself how much further work she would like to do to develop that particular skill. This is the essence of *experiential learning*.

Experiential learning

Experiential learning takes place when the students are given the opportunity to experience certain activities for themselves in a particular situation. The person who leads the activity can be a teacher, sister, staff nurse of nurse manager whose role it is to enable the student to experience the activity and draw conclusions from the experience.

This type of teaching/learning strategy is different from traditional teaching methods. Traditional teaching methods in classroom or wards begin with the predetermined end result 'By the end of this session the student will be able to do . . .' The teacher determines what this end result will be and the teaching session is geared to achieving it.

Experiential teaching methods do not work in this way. Instead, the student begins with her present level of achievement or ability in a certain skill. The teacher provides an activity, exercise or game which allows the student to develop that skill. The activity is such that it can cater for a wide range of skill levels within the group, and is chosen for the particular skill which is being developed at the time. The student controls the depth to which she wishes to work and then is helped by the teacher to explore, through discussion after the activity, what the activity felt like, what she learned from the activity and how she wishes further to develop that particular skill. The experience will be different for each student. Control over much of the content of the activity moves away from the teacher (as in traditional teaching) and is given to the student. In short, there is no predetermined end result from the teacher before she plans the teaching session. Her role is to provide an activity or exercise and let the student do with it what she wishes. The role and relationship between student and teacher changes when experiential teaching methods are used with a sharing of responsibilities and decision-making.

The direct, supported, personal experiencing of a situation, activity or exercise by a student practising a care planning skill enables her to become aware of how she felt in the experience, how skilled she feels in the situation and what further development she wishes for herself.

Much of this will not be new to some nurses, managers and teachers. What has been missing from our teaching programmes on care planning skills, however, is the structured use of experiential methods which allow students to discover where their skill strengths and weaknesses lie and how they can develop systematically these very sophisticated skills.

Let's throw away our fears!

Many teachers are worried about using experiential teaching methods and, undoubtedly, clinical nursing staff will be equally anxious when asked to teach students in this way. Many of these fears and anxieties are related to the fact that teachers, by and large, have had no training in using such methods, or they have used them so infrequently as not to feel skilled in their use. One step might be to undertake short courses in the use of experiential teaching methods (see Appendix).

Part of the process of feeling comfortable in using these techniques is to become more aware and accepting of one's own strengths and weaknesses, to be able to understand that it is all right to feel unconfident in this new way of teaching, to share this anxiety with colleagues and even students, and to 'take the plunge' by beginning to use one or two very simple experiential exercises or games, knowing that it is all right to learn even as your students are learning. If a teacher of clinical nurse permits herself to learn at the same time, this will diminish anxiety and the experience will become a learning one for all, teacher and taught alike.

One suggestion is that schools of nursing should consider employing, even as a temporary measure, teachers skilled in the use of experiential methods who can, in the first instance, take charge of some of the care planning skills development. Inviting other teachers to participate in their activities with students enables the less experienced teacher to begin to feel more comfortable with these methods, having watched a skilled person using them. These specialist teachers can serve as resource people for experiential methods, providing suggestions for appropriate games, activities and exercises for specific care planning skills development and organising workshops for teachers and ward staff who wish to develop their skills in using these teaching methods.

Another suggestion is for teachers and ward staff to come together on a regular basis as a support group for each other. Such group meetings can provide an opportunity for teachers and nurses to try out various experiential activities on their own colleagues in a relatively safe environment. It is an ideal time for teachers and nurses to share ideas, successes, failures, strengths and weaknesses in their use of experiential teaching methods.

The remainder of the book will provide useful resources for teachers and nurses who wish to try some fo these techniques for helping students develop care planning skills.

A word of warning!

Many teachers perceive experiential teaching methods as being synonymous with 'role play'. Role play is merely one form of experiential teaching which is, in fact, often used inappropriately or badly. There are a great many other forms of experiential activity which are far less threatening, and are certainly easier and more appropriate to use. Many teachers try to use role play, and indeed many other techniques, without ensuring first of all that they have the necessary skill and understanding of the technique. As role play has been mentioned, it is appropriate to use this particular teaching method to highlight problems which can arise when it is used indiscriminately or by an unskilled teacher. Firstly, role play is often perceived as being something which has to be done in front of a large audience or before a video camera: as a result this may cause students' anxiety levels to rise, often unnecessarily. Often, all the student learns in this situation is how unpleasant role play can be. Role play can take place without either audience or video camera and still have meaning as a learning experience. A student can play out a situation with another person which, given the appropriate follow-up and opportunity to reflect on what she has learned, will enable her to gain a personal insight into a particular situation and to develop the skills to manage it. Once the student is comfortable in this type of role play, observers or video can be introduced to provide the student with additional feedback.

A second misuse of role play involves the practice of 'de-roling' or 'de-briefing'. At the end of a role play activity, those who played roles should with the help of the teacher, have the opportunity to leave the role behind and all the feeling associated with being in the role, and come back to the present time to be themselves again. The phrase often used to describe de-roling is 'coming out of the role'. There are many effective ways of helping people de-role after a role play (see Appendix) and most of them are fairly simple procedures. When de-roling is not allowed, the students can take the feelings, emotions and thoughts of the role and the role play situation with them, which can cause anger, unhappiness, stress and other emotions to remain inside them rather than be left behind. Omitting to allow students to de-role can cause unresolved feelings to outweigh anything good that may have been gained from the role play.

Some words of caution are appropriate here. Firstly, as the teacher or facilitator of the activity, know what it is about, and understand how to use it well even if you are a little uncomfortable or inexperienced in using it. Ignorance can be a dangerous thing. Secondly, decide carefully on your *intention* when selecting a particular experiential activity. Why do you wish to provide that particular learning experience? Your answer should be 'I wish to allow the student to experience . . .' Then ask yourself whether or not the activity you have chosen will facilitate the intended process. Is there anything which may impede or prevent the student from participating in the activity? How can I minimise or alleviate this? Will a different learning experience serve the same purpose yet be free from any impediments to learning?

The process of learning from experience—or from an experiential activity—is a deliberate and conscious process which ultimately must involve allowing the student to reflect upon the activity or experience and herself derive meaning from it—to puzzle out from the experience what has happened to her and what and how she would like to develop in the future.

All experts on the subject of experiential learning agree that it is a cyclical process. One model which represents this process can be seen in Fig. 2.1; although this one was devised by the author, it is similar to those described by Pfeiffer & Jones (1982), Kilty (1982) and Bond (1982).

It shows that the experiential activity is not an end in itself—it is only the first part of a cyclical process of learning. It is the means by which some kind of learning can take place. The experience is used to enable the student to identify what it was like for her to have experienced such a situation, how she felt and how she reacted or percieved it. Through discussion, the dynamics of the experience are explored and applied to the real world. Lastly, but perhaps most importantly, the student must have the opportunity to determine explicitly how she might use what she has learned from the experience in future practice, such as in care planning, and what further learning experiences she wishes to undergo to develop further the particular skill or skills.

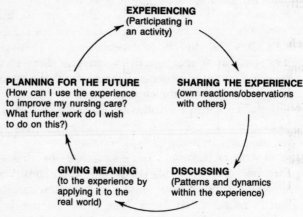

Fig. 2.1 Experiential learning cycle

Summary

Care planning involves many personal and interpersonal skills which can be taught or facilitated by teachers and clinical nurses both in school and at the bedside. Experiential teaching activities are the most appropriate teaching methods to use to enable students to develop these care planning skills.

Heath (1983) poignantly points out that the nurse has to survive in the ward situation. Acquiring coping skills is not enough: a good nurse needs to develop empathic skills and must be flexible and creative, know her strengths and weaknesses, and develop confidence in her abilities. How this happens will provide a link in the chain of her own development and the key to this link lies in the teaching methods employed by both teachers and clinical nurses to enable her to develop a wide range of skills. The most appropriate methods for teaching care planning skills are those of experiential teaching. The subject of experiential teaching methods has been introduced in this chapter, and the remainder of the book offers practical advice and suggestions about some of the activities which might be employed.

References

Bond M (1982) Cycle of experiential learning as described by Kilty, J in *Experiential Learning*. Human Potential Research Project, University of Surrey, p.5

Heath J (1983) Gaming/simulation in nurse education. *Nurse Education Today*, 3 (4), 92–5

Kilty J (1982) *Experiential Learning*. Guildford: Human Potential Research Project, University of Surrey

Pfeiffer J & Jones J (1982) *A Handbook of Structured Learning Experiences for Human Relations Training* Vol I. San Diego: University Associates

Chapter 3

Experiential Teaching Methods for Care Planning Skills: an Overview

Learning can take place in many ways. This chapter will concentrate on some of the learning activities which are particularly appropriate to the development of the care planning skills outlined in Chapter 1. They are also strategies which are most congruent with the experiential learning cycle (Fig. 2.1).

Care planning skills can be learnt at various levels in a variety of ways, all of which involve a wide range of activities which can be seen along a continuum represented in Fig. 3.1 as a straight line.

Low personal
involvement

High personal
involvement

Fig. 3.1   A continuum of learning activities

Low involvement is reactive learning where there is passive receiving of information. At the other end of the continuum, *high involvement* is an extreme interactive mode where students take total responsibility for, and guide, their own learning. Learning takes place through personally experiencing a situation or activity.

It is a simple exercise to take the continuum represented in Fig. 3.1 and put in specific learning activities where they might be found along it (see Fig. 3.2).

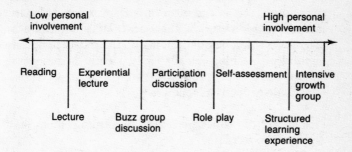

Fig. 3.2 Individual learning activities on the continuum

Another continuum which runs in parallel to the first one can be added to explain what type of learning experiences each of these activities is (see Fig. 3.3).

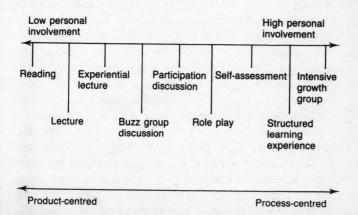

Fig. 3.3 The relationship between learning activities, high/low involvement and product/process orientation

The changing focus of teaching: towards process-centred teaching methods

When a school plans a curriculum, or when a teacher organises specific teaching sessions within that curriculum, one of the most important points is for the teacher to be aware of the particular programme or teaching session before deciding on the most appopriate method of teaching (Heath 1982). Heath defines these aims as being either product -centred or process-centred, which she explains as follows:

Product-centred concerned with informing them and giving them facts.

Process-centred concerned with helping students learn how to inform themselves; a concern with the process of development.

The content of a teaching session which is product- or process-centred might easily be the same, e.g. taking a nursing history, but the intention (aim) and the teaching methods will be very different. A product-centred session on how to take a nursing history will consist of imparting factual information about what a nursing history is and why it is important: a lecture or a discussion might be the method chosen. A process-centred session on the same subject will, however, involve learning activities which enable the student to take a nursing history in the relative safety of the classroom, perhaps with a colleague playing the part of a patient. The student will have the opportunity to reflect on her performance, learning from the experience of doing it. Equally, the student taking the role of the patient provides feedback to the student on her performance and how it felt being asked certain questions and so forth. In either case, the content of the session is the same but on one hand, the intention is for the student to gain knowledge (product-centred), while on the other hand, the intention is to experience and 'feel' what it is like to take a history (the process-centred approach). If the intention is that the student should have a sound theoretical knowledge and understanding of nursing histories, a product-centred teaching method will be the most appropriate. If, however, it is intended that the student should feel what it is like to take a history and to practise different ways of asking questions or making observations, then a process-centred teaching method is most appropriate. Heath (1982), in fact, identifies ways by which teachers can determine whether their teaching methods match their intentions. In terms of care planning knowledge and skills, a balanced programme is one which has the right mix of intentions and teaching methods for teaching both the knowledge and skills of care planning. The need for this balance and integration of the two approaches is further highlighted by the fact that product-centred teaching is concerned primarily with lower order cognitive skills, while process-centred teaching is concerned with the continual development of higher-level skills such as decision-making, problem-solving and interpersonal skills. Heath (1983) points out that the terms 'lower level' and 'higher level' skills do not suggest that one is more important than the other. Indeed, it is impossible for anyone to move to higher level skills without first having developed lower level ones. It is the correct balance between the two levels which is so essential and which allows nurses to learn the factual knowledge about care planning and then to experience the development of higher order care planning skills.

A nurse or teacher wishing to organise a teaching session related to care planning might use Fig. 3.2 or 3.3 to determine which teaching methods would be most appropriate for that session. The particular learning activities outlined in Fig. 3.2 are explained in greater detail, as follows:

Reading This is a low-involvement, product-centred activity whereby the student passively takes in facts or information with no need to become involved in any way with the material.

Lecture A lecture is a didactic information exchange session with minimal interpersonal involvement required between student and lecturer. Facts are passed on from a so-called 'expert' to a group of people seeking facts or information.

Experiential lecture This is a phrase used by Pfeiffer & Jones (1983) to describe a session which involves more than the traditional lecture and includes activity by the audience. The lecturer intersperses brief interactional activities throughout the lecture to allow the audience to experience for themselves some of the lecturer's ideas or to prepare the audience for the next topic within the lecture.

Discussion: buzz group This is a popular teaching strategy where small groups share ideas, information or opinions about a subject.

Participation discussion This is an extension of the discussion or buzz group because rather than only sharing ideas and information, feelings are shared as well. This strategy is often used to help students become more effective group members.

Role play This is a teaching strategy where the participants act out a sitation through parts which are assigned to them. These they attempt to play spontaneously by involving themselves wholly in the situation and trying to feel the part which they are playing. Another form of role play is self-role play or psychodrama, where one or more students play themselves in a particular situation which they have already experienced in real life but which they would like to learn to manage differently or understand better. In psychodrama, other students are assigned roles in the situation to help the student playing herself re-create the experience as it happened.

Self-assessment This is a learning strategy which allows the student to carry out certain activities, e.g. keeping a personal journal, to enable her to monitor her own performance and development.

Structured learning experience These learning activities are designed to enable students to focus on their own behaviour in a variety of settings using the experiential cycle described in Fig. 2.1. They can be used with various group sizes and are suitable for developing all the care planning skills described in Chapter 1. They can be used on their own or as part of an experiential lecture (see above). Activities which make up structured learning experiences are games, simulations, warm-up exercises, interpersonal activities, fantasy, human sculpting and many, many more.

Intensive group growth This is a very advanced type of experiential activity usually reserved for self-help or therapeutic encounter groups rather than for teaching in a nursing situation. It is characterised by very high personal involvement in the activity or group process.

One important point to recognise is that the further one travels from left to right along the continuum, the greater the amount of personal involvement and interaction required of both teacher and student and the greater the amount of self-disclosure and risk-taking by participants. The activities most appropriate for the development of care planning skills fall into three of the above categories: role play, self-assessment and structured learning experiences. Examples of how specific activities and exercises can be used both in the classroom and at the bedside will be found throughout the remainder of the book.

Summary

Learning from experience can take place in many ways. Experiential learning is very appropriate for developing the wide range of care planning skills identified in Chapter 1. This chapter has identified a continuum which shows the wide range of teaching methods available and identifies which of these teaching methods are most appropriate for helping students to develop care planning skills.

References

Heath J (1982) Intention and practice in nursing education. *Nurse Education Today*, **2** (4), 9–10

Heath J (1983) Gaming/simulation in nursing education. *Nurse Education Today*, **3** (4), 92–5

Pfeiffer J & Jones J (1983) *A Handbook of Structured Experiences for Human Relations Training*, Vol IX. San Diego: University Associates

Chapter 4

A Model for Helping: Six-category Intervention Analysis

The different schools of psychology and human behaviour offer various ways of describing how people relate to and interact with one another. No one model of interpersonal behaviour is necessarily better than another and some will be more understandable and meaningful to certain people than to others. In terms of nursing, the model of interpersonal behaviour chosen will form part of the framework for the way care planning skills are taught and should reflect the overall value and belief system of the school of nursing and health district.

Why have a model for teaching interpersonal skills?

A model of nursing is a pictorial representation of a theory, or the themes, ideas or beliefs about what nursing is; it also explains the relationship between nurse and patient and justifies the various aspects of the role and function of the nurse. A model of nursing determines what aspects of a patient's condition and circumstances it is important to assess when he is admitted and how the nurse should plan appropriate nursing care. Various authors have written about the models they have devised (eg. Orem 1971; Roper *et al*. 1985) and the nursing journals have published many articles on how to use models.

29

An excellent overview of nursing models in relation to the nursing process is found in Hunt & Marks-Maran (1986) and the practical application of models in various situations is covered in Kershaw & Salvage (1986).

A model will also explain where interpersonal skills development fits into nursing: how interpersonal skills development is approached must therefore reflect, or be compatible with, the nursing model employed. Examination of different frameworks for teaching interpersonal skills has identified some that are applicable to all nursing models or, indeed, apply even if no overt nursing model is used. One model of interpersonal skills which seems to be compatible with all schools of communication and nursing models of nursing is 'six-category intervention analysis' (Heron 1985). Despite its seemingly wordy title, this way of looking at interpersonal behaviour can be applied to nurse–nurse, nurse–patient and nurse–doctor relationships, or to any other interpersonal activity inside or outside nursing.

What is Six-category Intervention Analysis?

Six-category intervention analysis is a way of explaining and understanding how people relate and respond to one another. Stated simply, it means that all worthwhile interactions can be classified into one of six categories described by Heron:

Prescriptive intervention gives advice, judges, criticises or evaluates; in other words, seeks to direct the behaviour of another person.

Informative intervention gives instructions or information, interprets; seeks to impart new knowledge to another person.

Confronting intervention challenges, gives direct feedback: is intended to challenge a restrictive attitude, belief or behaviour of another person.

These three are called *authoritative* interventions because the helper, e.g. the nurse, takes a more overtly dominant role in the interaction and is intending to do so when interacting with the other person.

Cathartic intervention releases tension and encourages emotional outbursts such as anger, laughter or crying; seeks to enable another person to discharge an emotion.

Catalytic intervention allows the person to reflect on his behaviour; encourages the person to solve a problem for himself; seeks to enable a person to learn by self-discovery.

Supportive intervention approves, confirms, validates; seeks to affirm the person's worth and value.

These last three interventions are called *facilitative* interventions because the role of the helper, e.g. the nurse, is less obtrusive, more discreet and seeks to increase the patient's own self-awareness.

The word *intervention* is an unfortunate one and can be misunderstood and misinterpreted. For the sake of clarification, the word *interaction* can be used synonymously with intervention.

Most interactions between nurse and patient may be, in reality, a combination of several categories. Indeed, Heron himself says that supportive interventions must be a part of any and every helping situation. But using this model, all day-to-day interactions can be broken down and examined to see what type they are, whether alternative interactions are more appropriate, what effect different interactions might have on other people and which particular type of intervention each nurse favours or requires assistance to use more appropriately. Six-category intervention analysis provides a framework for each nurse to identify strengths and weakness in day-today interactions. Additionally, a wide variety of experiential teaching methods can be used to enable nurses to develop their skill in the use of each of the six categories of interventions.

It might be helpful to explore each of the six categories a little more closely.

Prescriptive interventions These explicitly and intentionally seek to influence and direct a patient's behaviour. The criteria for valid prescriptive interventions are that they should be presented in such a way as to leave the patient free to accept or reject the advice, judgement or criticism offered and that the prescription from the nurse does not deny the patient the right to be self-determining. It is easy to offer advice or suggestions to patients but it is less common for patients to be allowed explicitly to reject the advice. Here is an example: how is a patient offered a bowl of water for a wash in bed? Is he asked beforehand if this is what he wants and when he wants it? Or does a nurse go up to his bed carrying the bowl of water almost as a command that now is the time for a wash? It is hard for a patient to be self-determining when presented with a bowl of water without any prior negotiation about when this wash is to take place. A valid prescriptive interaction between nurse and patient must always make the patient feel that he is under no obligation to accept that prescription. In addition, the prescription (advice, suggestion) must be given with underlying support and respect for the patient's dignity and right to say no. It also must be given in a way which is not accidental but planned to give him the option of refusal.

Informative interventions These seek to impart knowledge, facts and information. They must be relevant to the patient's perceived needs and are directly related to many care planning activities. There is a great deal of information which nurses are called upon to give to

patients in a variety of settings, including factual or practical information, imparting new knowledge or
interpreting information or behaviour. Care planning is a
two-way process which involves receiving information
from a patient, using it and giving information back to
him. Informative interventions, therefore, are used in a
wide variety of care planning situations including assessment, patient teaching and enabling patients to make
informed decisions about treatment and care.

Confronting interventions These interventions, or
interactions, directly challenge—in a supportive and
caring manner—restrictive attitudes, beliefs or
behaviours of another person. In terms of care planning
confrontation may be necessary if the patient allows his
own rigidities and defences to prevent him from
participating in his own health care. More importantly,
confronting interventions are necessary if nurses are to
develop well in order to be able to act as the patient's
advocate with other health care professionals. Confronting interventions are the basis for the development of
assertiveness. A nurse may at any time find herself in a
situation where she is required to confront a patient's
relatives, her colleagues or doctors but by developing the
ability to use confronting interventions she will be able to
manage these situations in a non-threatening, non-
aggressive way.

Cathartic interventions These interventions are
intended to facilitate the expression of emotions such as
anger, grief, fear or embarrassment that are often painful.
Heron (1985) believes that these interventions are the
least developed in nurses and yet, in terms of care planning, are extremely important in helping patients or
relatives who are distressed. Many nurses respond to
situations of distress in others by actively discouraging
the expression of emotions. A nurse who is skilled at
cathartic interventions will be able, with care and

sensitivity, to allow a distressed person to express the emotions (as tears, laughter, rage, and so forth) and enable that person to grow. Emotions which remain inside a person can prevent him from resolving conflicts and from coping with adversity. Cathartic interventions, and learning to use them, lend themselves well to experiential learning activities and, in the relative safety of a classroom, nurses under skilled guidance can learn to deal comfortably with patients' emotions. Heron outlines a number of sorts of cathartic intervention and suggests learning activities to help nurses and others develop this skill (Herons 1985).

Catalytic interventions These are intended to help a patient or client grow, develop or solve a problem through self-discovery. The role of the nurse when using a catalytic intervention is to help this self-discovery take place through a variety of interpersonal strategies including the use of free attention, open questioning, self-disclosure and so forth. In terms of care planning, these skills are ideal in assessing patients' understanding of their illness and in helping them prepare for discharge and the future. Developing the ability to help others solve problems rather than always providing them with one's own opinion is one of the most important interpersonal skills which a nurse can acquire.

Supportive interventions This sixth type of interaction aims intentionally at affirming the worth of another person and is a method of telling someone that he has value. Supportive interventions are non-judgemental and unqualified: they are authentic and caring and are a way of letting a patient know that he is valued and respected and that the nurse is on his side. The kinds of supportive intervention which nurses can and should be developing include touch, expressing positive feelings, discreet self-disclosure and empathy. All care planning activities and all interpersonal situations must have an element of support in them.

Some final words about the six categories

It is important to realise that no one category is necessarily 'better' than another. Each category, when used appropriately, has great worth and value. Nurses appear to be better at using prescriptive, informative and supportive interventions than they are at using cathartic, catalytic and confronting ones (Heron 1985). Despite this, work by Hayward (1975), McLeod-Clark (1981) and others shows that even in the area of information-giving, nurses do not always do it well.

There appears to be a direct relationship between being skilled in the appropriate use of the six categories of intervention and developing good care planning skills. To be skilled at listening (giving free attention), observing, questioning and so forth, as well as in problem-solving, decision-making and in all the other care planning skills, involves an enormous amount of personal and interpersonal growth and development. The absence of structured activities which enable nurses to develop in this way seems to be a reason why care planning has not developed as much as it should. Six-category intervention analysis provides a framework by which the necessary personal and interpersonal skills can be developed and then applied to care planning. A variety of experiential activities (role play, self-assessment, structured learning experiences) can be employed to help nurses develop the ability to use and be comfortable with each type of intervention.

From six-category to care planning

Heron's six-category interventional analysis is an ideal way for nurses to identify and develop the interpersonal skills required to assess, plan and evaluate nursing care effectively. After breaking down the stages of care planning described in Chapter 1 into the skills required for each stage, appropriate learning activities can be organised to help nurses to become more able to use all the interventions well. If one examines the skills required to assess patients, one identifies a number of categories of intervention which are required for effective patient assessment. Six-category interventional analysis provides a framework for self-assessment by nurses of their own areas of strengths and weakness with regard to the interpersonal skills required to assess, plan and evaluate care.

Summary

Six-category intervention analysis is one framework for developing the interpersonal skills necessary to plan and give individualised nursing care. It is congruent with all models of nursing and provides a way for nurses to identify areas of strength and weakness and to develop the skills of interaction which are required to meet people's needs effectively.

References

Hayward J (1975) *Information: a Prescription Against Pain*. London: RCN

Heron J (1985) *Six Category Intervention Analysis*. Guildford: University of Surrey, Department of Educational Studies

Hunt J & Marks-Maran D (1986) *Nursing Care Plans: the Nursing Process at Work*. Chichester: John Wiley & Sons

Kershaw B & Salvage J (1986) *Models for Nursing*. Chichester: John Wiley & Sons

McLeod-Clark J (1981) Communication in nursing: analysing nurse-patient conversations. *Nursing Times*, **77** (1), 12–18

Orem D (1971) *Nursing: Concepts of Practice*. New York: McGraw Hill

Roper N Logan W & Tierney A (1985) *The Elements of Nursing*. Edinburgh: Churchill Livingstone

Section II

Chapter 5

Skills for Assessing Patients

The process of assessing patients involves many of the interpersonal skills described in Chapter 1, including observing, listening, questioning, supporting, self-disclosing, reflecting and trust-building. This list is not exhaustive—many skills can be identified and in reality there is tremendous overlap between many of them. However, in order to be able to teach and develop these skills they need to be presented as individual skills to be practised, polished and developed individually so that, when they are brought together in assessing a patient, the combination of skills will result in a good assessment. Some teachers refer to this as the 'gymnasium principle'. An athlete who is a marathon runner, for example, will spend time in the gymnasium exercising each of the separate muscles of his body. If one were to watch this athlete in training and see him spend an hour just exercising his biceps, one might ask 'What does this biceps exercise have to do with running a marathon?' The answer is that each of his muscles has to be fully and individually developed so that arms, legs, neck, trunk, back and diaphragm eventually are individually in tiptop shape so that on the day of the race, they will work together in perfection.

Each separate interpersonal skill is like the separate muscles of an athlete's body. Each skill must be practised to perfection separately so that when they are all brought together they work in unison in the best possible way.

The teacher or ward nurse can apply the gymnasium principle to the activities she provides to enable her students to develop each component part of interpersonal skills and, ultimately, to practise patient assessment with ease, skill and confidence. One other function of teaching interpersonal skills by separating the various components is that this heightens the nurse's awareness of areas of assessment which can so easily be overlooked, ignored or missed.

Communication

Students enter nursing believing that they know how to communicate. After all, they have been doing it all their lives, haven't they? Research with nurses, however, shows that this is not necessarily the case (McLeod-Clark 1981; Bridge & Speight 1981). The hardest task that a teacher or ward sister can have is to help students to realise that there are different levels and ways of communicating and that the skills required to communicate with friends, family and acquaintances in everyday social life are very different from those they require as nurses. Communicating with people in a helping, professional capacity involves highly complex interpersonal skills; the breaking down of these into their component parts and the provision of activities to practise and develop each part enable students to develop the level of professional communication required of them.

Interpersonal skills for assessment

Assessment is the continuous process of collecting information from patients which nurses need to plan and give appropriate care. Some of the skills required to assess patients were identified in the opening paragraph of this chapter and of these, the following will be explored in greater depth:

- Observing
- Listening
- Questioning

The other skills identified at the start of this chapter also lend themselves to assessment but will be discussed later in Section III.

A nursing history is a valuable tool in the collection of information but requires an interaction between two people. This interaction must be a comfortable one for both the people involved. La Monica (1985) suggests that pre-planning an interview with a patient is an important method of examining some of the interactions which could arise during a nursing history and whether or not a nurse will feel comfortable with them if they should arise. The following is an example of a pre-planning interview exercise.

EXERCISE

The student undertaking this exercise is given the following information:

'You are a 19-year-old student nurse working your first week on a medical ward. Mr James, a 46-year-old accountant suffering from angina, is admitted to the ward. It is his first admission to hospital and you have been asked to admit him and take a nursing history. You know a fair amount about angina as you learned about it in your last study block. You go to his bedside, and find him lying on the bed reading a newspaper. His colour and breathing appear quite good and he seems comfortable. You introduce yourself and tell him that you would like to ask him some questions so that you can plan the best nursing care for him. You begin the interview. All is going well until you ask him when he first noticed the chest pain. He hesitates, looks uncomfortable and says (hurriedly) that it was when he was making love to his wife.'

Questions to ask yourself:

- Is this an important point to pursue?
- Do you require further information about it?
- What questions might be going through your mind?
- Are you comfortable in this situation?
- Can you deal with it?
- Are you able to ease his discomfort and embarrassment?

These questions can form the basis of discussion between nurses working in pairs, small groups or with a large class. Role play might be used to act out the situation.

Variations

Another activity could be substituted for the activity which triggered the angina to see if the same, or different, problems arise.

This exercise is one of any number of activities which can be used to pre-plan a nursing history interview and to anticipate difficult inter-personal situations that may arise during the interview. Students can be encouraged to keep a record of interesting, difficult or uncomfortable nursing history interview situations which they encounter and which can be used in future teaching sessions. By anticipating situations, the nurse can ask herself 'Do I have the knowledge, experience and ease to deal with this type of question?' If the answer is 'no' she has then identified a skill area which she now knows she needs to develop. By identifying such uncomfortable interview situations or questions, the nurse can do two things

- She can ask a teacher, sister or more experienced nurse to come with her as she takes a particular nursing history which might prove to be difficult for her.
- She can role play the situation with friends or colleagues and then use the experiential cycle (Fig. 2.1) to plan how she can use the role play for future practice.

An experienced teacher or ward sister knows that certain interview situations—perhaps the one described in the above exercise—will arise time and time again. Some more senior nurses have the ammunition of experience to deal with these situations, but the less experienced nurse can learn by using critical incidents as a way of identifying and anticipating difficulties, and plan ways of coping with them.

The first step, therefore, in assessing patients is to develop the feeling of being comfortable with whatever situation might arise: this happens through the acquisition of knowledge and skill in the relative safety of a learning activity with support and guidance from a teacher or experienced nurse.

Observation skills

Intelligent observation begins with knowledge. Although a nurse can observe a patient with little knowledge of his illness, knowing particular facts about the illness will give specific guidelines to what she should look for. Nurses can do a great deal to enhance and develop their ability to observe well. Observation begins with heightening awareness about something: many exercises are available for increasing nurses' ability to be aware of what is around them. Here is one.

EXERCISE

This exercise is called 'Now I am aware'.

Working in pairs students spend two to five minutes quietly talking to each other, beginning each sentence with the phrase 'Now I am aware of . . . .' Each completes the sentence with something she is aware of at that moment—something she hears, sees, feels, thinks about that is going on around or within her.

Examples of 'Now I am aware' sentences include:

- Now I am aware of the bird singing outside.
- Now I am aware that my tummy is rumbling.
- Now I am aware that you are smiling.

After undertaking this exercise, each nurse should be given the opportunity to talk about how she felt doing the exercise and what the exercise was like for her.

Exercises such as this one can help to increase nurses' awareness of what is going on around them. Discussion can follow about the kinds of thing they can become aware of in their day-to-day work with patients.

A sensitive teacher or ward sister can turn day-to-day interactions with students into awareness-raising strategies by asking them after an interaction or patient situation 'What are you thinking (or feeling, or noticing) right now?' Equally, a teacher can use her own observation of how a student behaves to heighten the nurse's own awareness of how inner feelings can be demonstrated by her behaviour. For example, the teacher might say to a nurse 'You seem to be tense' or 'I see you are stressed. What are you feeling?'

By becoming aware of one's own tensions and how they are observed by others one can begin to be more aware of one's own feelings and to be more observant and perceptive of how others behave. This self-awareness is a basic prerequisite for many more complex activities such as problem-solving and decision-making. Observing ourselves also enables us to observe others more sensitively. Once students become more sensitive to their own feelings and behaviour, the time will have come to undertake observation activities specifically related to patients. One simple but effective ward-based observation exercise is called 'The Observation Game'.

EXERCISE: THE OBSERVATION GAME

The teacher selects several patients, tells her students who she has selected and gives the students three minutes to walk round the ward observing and remembering everything they can about those patients. The teacher then calls the students together and asks specific questions about the selected patients. A point is given to whoever first gives the correct answer.

Examples of questions

Which patient has the blue dressing gown? Which patient has peripheral cyanosis? In which arm is Mr Smith's infusion?

Many nurses are well aware of body language and how powerful messages can be transmitted non-verbally through gesture, facial expression, posture and touch. Sometimes, however, nurses lack the skills required to check that the non-verbal messages they receive from a patient are in fact the same messages that he is sending. Checking is an important component in understanding non-verbal communication and the following exercise is intended especially for developing skills in observing non-verbal communication.

EXERCISE

Purpose of exercise:

To become aware of how different emotions can be expressed non-verbally and to validate one's perception of non-verbally expressed emotions.

This exercise is best carried out with students sitting round a large table or in a circle, and takes about 30–40 minutes. The ideal group size is twelve to fifteen but larger groups can split into smaller ones.

How to play

Each student is invited to write down on a small piece of paper an emotion or feeling. These papers are folded in half and put into a basket. On a second piece of paper, each student is invited to write down a part of the body which can be used to express a feeling or emotion, and these papers are folded in half and placed in a second basket. Each student then picks one slip of paper from each basket and is asked to act out the emotion selected using the body part she has also selected. Every other member of the group tries to guess what feeling or emotion is being acted out. All members of the group should have the chance to act out a feeling, and discussion should follow focusing on what the students have learned from the exercise. This discussion can take place after each nurses's turn at acting out or on completion of the entire exercise.

These are only a very small sample of the wide range of exercises which can help students to develop their ability, awareness and skill related to observing people. Please refer to the end of the chapter for references to other exercises.

Listening

Listening is not the same thing as hearing. We listen in

many ways and different types of listening are appropriate to different situations. Heron (1985) uses the term *free attention* instead of listening as a skill for supportive and catalytic interventions. He says that free attention implies something much more than social listening and describes free attention as:

> '. . . the practitioner (nurse) giving all his (her) available attention, that is, all his attention that is not distracted by other events in the environment and that is not distracted inwards by his own psychological noise—negative thoughts, feelings and pre-occupations.'

What Heron is saying is that in our attempts to listen to people we are consciously or unconsciously interrupted by events and distractions going on either around us or inside us. On the ward, this might be the rattling of the tea trolley or our own rumbling tummy as we become aware that it is nearly lunch time. Heron says that free attention is a subtle yet extremely powerful and intense activity of being completely with the patient and tuned in to the patient. Free attention uses posture, gaze, facial expression and touch.

Using the 'Now I am aware' exercise described earlier, it is easy to realise just how often, and insidiously, internal and external happenings prevent us from giving free attention. The following is a simple exercise which any nurse can carry out during a spare few minutes at work. The exercise will help raise awareness about internal and external distractions which prevent us from giving free attention.

EXERCISE

Sit down at the nurse's desk in your ward. Select *one* thing which is going on either in the ward around you or inside you. Make it a point to concentrate totally only on that thing which you have selected (e.g. the beating of your heart, or Mrs Smith in bed 6). Do this for three minutes. When this time is up note all the things which distracted you whilst you were trying to give free attention to your chosen subject.

Other suggestions for free attention exercises are given at the end of the chapter. Note that other writers on communication and interpersonal skills use the term 'active listening' to mean the same thing as giving free attention (Egan 1986; Pfeiffer & Jones 1974–1983).

Questioning skills

We use many kinds of question in our everyday social interaction and in our professional lives. In terms of care planning, skilled questioning is required to elicit the most appropriate information from patients in order to maximise our assessment of them. Questions are categorised in two ways: closed and open questions.

What is meant by closed and open questions?   Closed questions are those which can be answered by 'yes' or 'no' and in some cases are questions whose answer is already known or assumed by the questioner, e.g. 'You're feeling better today, aren't you?' Closed questions are, for the most part, worded so that the patient is neither invited nor encouraged to expand on the information. There is a place for closed questions in certain assessment situations, although many communication purists would argue against this. In any event, closed questions take less time to ask and to answer and people generally feel more comfortable with them.

An open question, on the other hand, is one which invites an informative response from the patient. In fact, the question which forms the heading of this subsection is an example of an open question. Some authors, (e.g. Heron 1985) use the term 'client-centred question' instead of open question to mean the same thing. When a question is client-centred it enables the patient to elaborate on thoughts, feelings and information in greater depth if he so chooses. This not only gives information to the questioner but, more importantly, gives the patient himself an insight into a situation or happening in his life. An open question does not point the way to *what* the patient might discover—rather, it just allows the patient freedom to discover or disclose as much or as little as he chooses. Open, client-centred questions in an assessment interview tell the patient that the nurse is really interested in what he thinks or feels and can, when carried out skilfully, enable him to discover a relationship between his illness and what is happening around and within him.

From the nurse's point of view, however, detailed and accurate information comes from asking open questions. The question 'How do you sleep at night?' will elicit more information useful in planning care than just asking 'Do you sleep well?' The latter is leading and only invites the patient to answer 'yes' or 'no'. There is no invitation to him to elaborate on what sleeping well means, how many hours of sleep he gets, and so on. An anxious patient might feel obliged to say he sleeps well because the closed question implies that this is the 'right' answer. The following exercise is a simple game to help students to develop their ability to ask different sorts of question and to note the differences in asking both open and closed questions.

EXERCISE

(Devised by Janice Scott and used with her permission.)

Materials

1   A pack of cards on each of which is written either the word 'closed' or 'open'. Have an equal number of each in the pack.

2   Another pack of cards each with a subject written
       on it. Subjects might include:

- What I did last weekend
- My favourite ward sister
- My sleep habits
- How I feel about nursing

and any other you may wish to choose.

Process

The group sits in a circle (twelve to fifteen people is the
ideal size). One student picks up the top card from the
stack of subject cards and shows it to the group. The
students on either side of her each take a card from the
'open' and 'closed' question pack and, without disclosing
what is on it, in turn ask a question related to the subject
yet which is representative of the type of question
indicated on their cards. The rest of the group guesses
what type of question it is. In addition, the receiver of the
questions, e.g. the person who selected the subject card,
answers both questions and afterwards, comments on
how it felt to be asked each question. The group can
discuss the types of questions used, the amount and
completeness of the answers and which type of question
seemed most appropriate to use in the situation.

A second exercise might be used to practise different
types of question and to observe the effects of using
them. A role play can be done in pairs, with a third
person acting as observer. The role play scenario can be a
nurse taking a history from a patient. After the role play
the two players can evaluate for themselves what it felt
like asking and answering different types of questions
and the observer can provide additional feedback by
discussing her observations with them. The teacher must
remember to allow the players to de-role or de-brief at the
end of the session (see Appendix). Further information

about the role of the observer can be found at the end of Chapter 9.

Conclusion

Assessing patients is a highly complex activity requiring a number of interpersonal skills. The three main skills are those of observing, listening and questioning, but woven through all three of them is the skill of supporting through non-verbal cues and tone of voice. Numerous teaching exercises have been suggested which can be used in classroom or ward-based teaching programmes. Other skills such as supporting, self-disclosure, trust-building and reflecting will play a part in assessing patients—these will be discussed in greater depth in later chapters.

References

Bridge W & Speight I (1981) Teaching the skills of communication, *Nursing Times* (Occasional Paper), **77** (32), 125–7

Egan G (1986) *The Skilled Helper.* Monterey: Brooks/Cole

Heron J (1985) *Six Category Intervention Analysis*, Guildford: University of Surrey, Department of Educational Studies

La Monica E (1985) *The Humanistic Nursing Process.* Boston: Jones & Bartlett

McLeod-Clark J (1981) Communication in nursing: analysing nurse-patient conversations. *Nursing Times*, **77** (1), 12–18

Pfeiffer J & Jones J (1974–1983) *A Handbook of Structured Experiences for Human Relations Training*, Vols I–IX. San Diego: University Associates

Additional exercises related to assessment skills

Brandes D (1982) *The Gamester's Handbook—II*. London: Hutchinson

Game no. A P 34, page 58—Attending-non-attending
This game is played in groups of four where one person is designated speaker and is asked to talk for one or two

minutes on a particular subject. A second person listens attentively (gives free attention or active listening) and a third person acts as a non-listener and deliberately avoids paying any attention to the speaker. The fourth player is an observer and carefully notes the behaviour of the other three. Everyone has the chance to play each role. Discussion follows which centres on how each felt in each role, what the observers saw was going on and what behaviour makes for 'good' attending. Variations of the game are also suggested by the author.

Pfeiffer J & Jones J (1974–1983) *A Handbook of Structured Experiences for Human Relations Training,* Vol I–IX. San Diego: University Associates

Pfeiffer & Jones have published a variety of exercises for various aspects of personal and interpersonal development. Many of them are particularly relevant for teaching the assessment skills described in Chapter 5. The reader is referred to the following exercises:

Handbook Vol. no.	Exercise no.	Page	Title/type of activity
1	8	31	Listening
1	22	101	Non-verbal communication
2	44	94	Non-verbal communication
3	52	10	Not listening
3	72	97	Non-verbal communication
5	152	13	Helping relationships
5	153	16	Babel
7	252	39	Active listening
7	257	73	Sunglow

La Monica E (1979) *The Nursing Process: a Humanistic Approach*. Menlo Park: Addison-Wesley

La Monica includes a variety of exercises for developing care planning skills. Two which are specifically related to assessing patients are:

- Personalised Care Plan (La Monica 1979, page 158)
- Nursing History Interview Format (La Monica 1979, page 165)

Chapter 6

Skills for Making Nursing Diagnoses and Planning Care

The skills for assessing patients described in the previous chapter apply to all stages of the care planning process as well as to assessment. Some other specific interpersonal skills are also particularly relevant to helping nurses to make nursing diagnoses and plan nursing care.

Making a nursing diagnosis involves cognitive understanding of the patient's illness and the disease process. It also involves an understanding of what is meant by a nursing diagnosis and how it differs from a medical diagnosis. Hunt & Marks-Maran (1986) offer definitions and explanations of what is meant by a nursing diagnosis and how to identify it. Briefly, the nursing diagnosis identifies the problems or unmet needs which a patient has (perceived by himself or the nurse) or which he might possibly have as a result of his illness or his personal and social situation: it is the reason why nursing care is required. The nursing diagnosis is arrived at by making sense out of all the assessment information and as such it is the next step in the problem-solving process. Concise identification of a problem—in this case we call it a nursing diagnosis—is important in order to determine how to solve the problem. The two main skills required to identify nursing diagnoses and to plan care are:

- Problem identification
- Setting priorities

What is the problem?

The nursing diagnosis has three parts: identification of the patient's actual or possible problem, the cause of the problem, and how the patient is behaving because of the problem. Therefore, learning activities must be provided for nurses so that they may develop the ability to identify all three parts.

The use of critical incidents—vignettes, case histories, real or created anecdotes or situations which arise in nursing practice—is an ideal way for students to identify actual and possible problems, either as written descriptions brought to the classroom or in the ward for teaching as they arise. In any event, they are realistic patient situations which the students can use, with guidance and facilitation from a teacher or ward sister, to discuss and plan how to identify the nursing diagnoses. Ideas can be shared on the nature and cause of the problems, how the patient behaves and, in the case of a possible problem, how they will notice that it is becoming an actual problem. Teaching methods for using these critical incidents might include many on the continuum of teaching activities described in Fig. 3.2, including buzz groups, discussion, and role play.

The use of critical incidents in conjunction with buzz groups or discussion enables students to identify how the patient might demonstrate that a problem—or possible problem—exists. Demonstration of a problem might occur in patients by any of the following means:

- Something the patient is saying ('I am in pain')
- Use of measurement tools (body pain chart, pain thermometer)
- Non-verbal behaviour (facial expression, rigid posture)
- Release of emotions (wailing, tears, moans)

Critical incidents or case studies can help nurses to develop cognitive insight into the problems of a patient and a wider understanding and feeling for the many different ways by which a patient demonstrates that he has a problem. Awareness of the reaction of a patient to his problems also provides a yardstick by which improvement can be measured.

As well as cognitive knowledge, critical incidents of the kind described above lend themselves to experiential activities, such as role play, which will enhance the nurse's ability to empathise with feelings which a patient experiences. The following are examples of learning activities related to the identification of nursing diagnoses.

EXERCISE 1

This is an activity similar to one described in the previous chapter which uses two packs of cards. The first pack has a particular nursing or patient problem written on each card, e.g. pain, anxiety, fear, depression and so on, while the second pack of cards contains various ways of assessing the problem, e.g. facial expression, immobility, emotional release, measurement tools, statement from a patient, and so on.

The exercise requires a group of up to ten participants. It can also be done in smaller groups of two or three.

Materials

Two packs of cards as described above.

Method

1   A participant chooses one card from each pack. Using the behaviour shown on the second card, she acts out the problem shown on the first card.
2   The rest of the group has to guess what the problem is from the behaviour being demonstrated.
3   Discussion can follow in which both the performer and the spectators share their feelings; the

performer on how it was to act out the situation and the spectators on how they felt watching the problem being demonstrated.

EXERCISE 2

This is a very simple role play. Using a case history or incident which has actually been encountered by someone in the group, a particular nursing problem is identified, e.g. pain. This is the situation upon which the role play is based.

Nurses can work in pairs or threes to role play with each other. One student plays the part of a nurse, another takes the part of the patient and the third person, if there is one, acts as observer.

Materials

None required.

Method

1   Using a critical incident or situation of a patient with a problem, e.g. pain, the pair or threesome discuss the situation for a few minutes—what may have caused the problem and how the patient behaved in relation to it.
2   The role play follows. The 'patient' demonstrates being in pain in any way she wishes (verbally or non-verbally). Using the interview and observation skills discussed in Chapter 5, the 'nurse' attempts to:
     (a)   identify and describe the patient's behaviour as it is being role played, and
     (b)   help the patient to describe the problem to her, using catalytic techniques as described in Chapter 4 and some of the strategies described in Chapter 5 (such as open-ended questions, reflection, free attention and touch).

3   After the role play (which takes as long as the players wish it to take) the two role players and the observer should discuss what happened, as follows:

(a)   The one playing the patient should reflect upon and describe what it was like being a person in pain and how it felt to be helped by the nurse to express her pain.

(b)   The nurse should then discuss how it was for her using the skills needed to help the patient express her pain.

(c)   Finally, the observer tells the others how it looked from her position. The observer should criticise the observation/interview skills of the nurse constructively and give praise as she wishes (see Chapter 10).

4   The participants should then repeat the same or another role play situation playing different roles and discussing the role play afterwards.

5   At the end of all the role play situations, de-roling (de-briefing) should be carried out by the teacher or group facilitator. Methods of de-roling and reasons why it is important are discussed in the Appendix.

A wide variety of other problem-solving activities can be found in Pfeiffer & Jones (1983), Brandes & Phillips (1977), Brandes (1982) and Burnard (1985).

Setting Priorities

Priority setting is a highly sophisticated skill that is essential to the placing of all nursing problems in some order of importance. It is a skill which is often difficult for junior nurses to acquire as they may not be aware of some of the nuances and implications of certain nursing diagnoses. Historically, patient priorities were determined by doctors' orders or medical needs: all nursing care is given in terms of doctors' needs, nurses' needs, and ward routines rather than individual patient problems placed in some order of priority (Hunt & Marks-Maran 1986).

The order in which nurses carry out nursing care reflects the value or importance placed on certain aspects of nursing care (this will be described in greater depth in Chapter 8). But if we truly believe that nursing care should be based on the priorities of each individual patient, it follows that nurses must have the opportunity to develop the skill of setting priorities from the total list of nursing diagnoses at any one time. As the list changes, as problems occur or are solved and as the patient's health status changes, so, too, will the priorities for patient care change. Fig. 6.1 shows the process by which priorities for nursing activities can be identified. By using Fig. 6.1, learning activities can be created which can be used to help nurses to examine any patient and his nursing diagnoses.

EXERCISE 3

This is a group activity which uses real patient information to help nurses to practise priority setting.

Materials

A nursing case history for each group of three or four nurses. The groups can explore the same case history but it is often more realistic if each group uses the history of a patient known to one or more of the members. A good amount of assessment information is given for each patient. The nursing diagnoses (problems, causes and demonstrated behaviours) can either be given in the case history or identified by the group as part of the exercise.

Method

1   Each group chooses its own case history or one is provided by the teacher. The value in the group

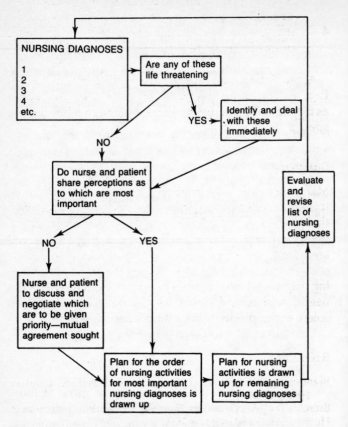

Fig. 6.1 Identifying the priorities for nursing activities

    choosing its own is that there is a certain amount of commitment and motivation when real situations known to the group are used.

2   Each group works through the case history, identifies nursing diagnoses (unless these have been given) and sets the diagnoses in order of priority, using Fig. 6.1 as a guideline.

3   The group can then draw up a plan for nursing care for that patient for one day: it can be done as a

structured care plan with diagnoses in order of priority or in a timetable format indicating what care will be given at what times during the day.

4 The group can discuss the activity with other groups to compare their plans or timetables.

A simulation game for priority setting entitled 'Front Page' will be found in Jones (1978) and can be used either as it is described in the book or modified to relate it more specifically to nursing.

Summary

Making a nursing diagnosis is a formal way of becoming totally aware of patient problems or possible problems, their causes and the behaviour being demonstrated by the patient as a result of his problems. The skills involved are, firstly, the identification of the problems and their components and, secondly, putting the problems (nursing diagnoses) into an order of priority which reflects the needs, wishes and desires of the patients rather than solely at the dictates of the doctor or nurse.

References

Brandes D & Phillips H (1978) *Gamester's Handbook*. London: Hutchinson

Brandes D (1982) *Gamester's Handbook II*. London: Hutchinson

Hunt J & Marks-Maran D (1986) *Nursing Care Plans: the Nursing Process at Work*. Chichester: John Wiley & Sons

Burnard P (1985) *Learning Human Skills*. London: Heinemann

Jones K (1978) Front page. In: Taylor & Walford (eds) *Learning and the Simulation Game*. Milton Keynes: Open University Press

Pfeiffer J & Jones J (1983) *A Handbook of Structured Experiences for Human Relations Training*, Vols I–IX. San Diego: University Associates

Chapter 7

Skills for Evaluating

The subject of how to evaluate care is relatively new to nursing. Although most nurses agree that there is a need to evaluate care, the task of actually carrying out evaluation is a complex one requiring clarification of what it is wished to evaluate as well as how to do it. Recently, attempts have been made to identify standards statements as criteria against which nursing care can be evaluated. La Monica (1979) points out, however, that several facets of care must be evaluated. These are:

- Restoring the patient to health, with his problems alleviated as defined in the nursing diagnosis
- Level of personal and professional growth of the care givers in relation to the skills and abilities necessary to give care
- Effectiveness of leadership style used in implementing the care

If we use these three components to evaluate nursing, we widen the scope of evaluation to include what happens to nurses as well as what happens to patients.

Evaluation by measuring outcomes against expectations

The most well-known, although not often formally

practised, method of evaluation is the behavioural approach whereby the nurse observes whether or not predetermined goals for patients have been achieved. It is best carried out by a group of nurses in a particular clinical setting (such as at a ward meeting) because the more people who are involved in the evaluation process, the more accurate will be the evaluation. Whenever nursing diagnoses are made, goals or aims of care can be set and some sort of evaluation can be carried out in terms of the extent to which the goals have been reached. Writing specific goals or expected outcomes for each nursing diagnosis can be used as the basis for formal evaluation at a future date or time. Less formal evaluation can also take place when no predetermined goals have been set by identifying the patient's response to the care he is being given. All too often, however, evaluation is unplanned and observations such as 'no pyrexia today' or 'appears less anxious' are made in an informal way and at the whim of the nurse. These informal methods of evaluation are those most often used by nurses in practice.

Nurses can be helped in several ways to learn more about the more formal, systematic evaluation of care, such as the use of outcome measures. One effective method of teaching the measurement of nursing care is through the use of critical incidents. Students are invited and encouraged at a teaching session to identify and describe incidents of patient care in which they have been involved. These may be positive or negative examples of the use of formal evaluation methods and the choice of the incident is left to the discretion of the individual nurse. Nurses work in pairs or small groups, taking a particular incident presented by one of the group and identifying what sort of evaluation method was used, whether outcomes of care were measured, what was present in, or omitted from, the care plan which either helped or hindered evaluation of care and how they could or might improve the evaluation situation in the future. The entire class can, if appropriate, discuss what they learnt through exploring their particular incidents. This type of teaching session can be carried out in the classroom or as part of a ward-based teaching session.

Evaluation by measurement of the personal and professional growth of the care giver

Evaluation can also be viewed in terms of the personal and professional growth of the nurse and can be measured in three ways: evaluation by her managers, evaluation by colleagues (peer evaluation) and self-evaluation. Evaluation by managers (ward sisters, nursing officers, tutors) tends to be the measurement which is given most importance in nursing, and is often punitive. It is the use of peer and self-assessment strategies, however, which should be encouraged as a way of learning about one's own performance in patient care and team membership.

Nurses can be stimulated to learn to evaluate their own performance in many ways. One is to encourage each nurse to keep a personal journal, which will provide her with her own continous record and assessment of her perception of her performance. In addition, every activity described in this and other chapters can end with a time for self-assessment to enable nurses who have engaged in the activity to reflect on how they carried it out, what they felt and what they have learned from it. There are many ways of helping nurses to evaluate their own performance in an experiential learning activity, two of which are described below.

SELF-ASSESSMENT ACTIVITY 1: 'BEST AND LEAST'

This is a self-assessment strategy by which individual nurses can identify what they liked best and least about their performance during a group learning activity. It can also be used by nurses to evaluate the teacher's performance as leader of the activity by identifying what they liked best and least about the way the activity was organised and led. The exercise can be done in a circle, with each member of the group taking it in turn to identify the thing she liked best about her performance (or the performance of the teacher) during the activity; it is followed by a round of what each nurse liked least. It is important that the teacher should make it clear that statements of best and least should be made thoughtfully and gently and in a supportive way. Equally, it must be made clear to all the participants that each nurse gives her best and least statement without comment, criticism or judgement from anyone else in the group.

SELF-ASSESSMENT ACTIVITY 2: 'ONE THING I HAVE LEARNED . . .'

This is a variation on the previous exercise.

Each student has the opporutnity to identify one thing she has gained or learned from a teaching session. This is often less threatening to the nurses as they are free to choose to tell the group whatever they wish: equally, they can choose not to share anything and merely say 'pass' when their turn comes to speak. As with the previous self-assessment activity, the nurses sit in a circle for the activity and no comment, criticism or judgement is made.

These two exercises are ways by which nurses can develop skills to evaluate what is going on around them the same skills that can be applied to the evaluation of nursing care. A particular ward sister known to the author uses the two self-assessment activities as a way of ending each work day or shift. Before sending her nurses home, she asks each one to identify what she thought was best about her nursing care that day and what she liked least. Alternatively, she asks each nurse as she goes off duty to identify one thing she had learnt that day.

As well as learning to evaluate oneself and one's own practice, an important evaluation skill that the nurse should develop is the ability to engage in group and peer evaluation. Groups of nurses can learn to evaluate the whole group's performance in a situation and reach mutually agreed conclusions. Group and peer evaluation can take place at the end of a learning session in which the group have worked together on a task; the skill acquired can be used by a group of nurses to evaluate their performance in working together to give nursing care. One way of helping nurses to build evaluation skills as a group and mutually to agree conclusions about the group's work is through the use of the 'nominal group technique'.

NOMINAL GROUP TECHNIQUE

This enables a group of people to draw conclusions about a group activity, which can be a classroom learning activity, entire study block or nursing care in a clinical area.

Method

1   Each nurse, working on her own, draws up a list of activities which she feels reflects what the group did best in some recent activity or set of activities, which might have been in the classroom or nursing care carried out by the group as a team.
2   Nurses then join together in groups of two or three to compare their individual lists and to compile a composite list which contains items on which they *all* agree.
3   The teacher then asks each group in turn to identify an item from their agreed composite list. This is written on a blackboard or large piece of paper for all groups to see. The teacher continues asking each group in turn and writing their responses until each

group is satisfied that all the items on their composite list now appear on the large list and the front of the room.

4 The teacher then asks if there are any individual personal items not already on the list which anyone would like to add to it.

5 The entire group is now left with a fairly long list of statements representing what is seen to be best about the group's work or activities. Each nurse is allocated ten votes. She can use these votes in any way she wishes. Working on her own, each nurse looks at the list of items and apportions her ten votes to the statements on the list. She can, for example, allocate one vote to each of ten statements if she feels there are ten items about which she feels equally strong. Alternatively, she can give all ten votes to one statement about which she feels strongly. She also has the option to give four votes to one statement, three votes to another, and so on.

6 The teacher then asks each nurse in turn to say what votes she has given. A tick is made next to each statement for each vote that statement receives. When all the nurses have given their votes, the total number of ticks for each statement is counted and recorded next to the statement. This gives a picture of how the group evaluates—as a group—what was best about a particular activity in which they have all engaged.

7 The exercise can be repeated with the group identifying what they liked *least* about a recent activity.

The nominal group technique is an extremely valuable way of allowing a group of people to evaluate their group work, their recent learning experiences or the nursing care they gave when working together as a team.

Self-evaluation and group evaluation are sophisticated skills for nurses to develop in their personal and professional lives. Care planning includes evaluation, and a part of such an evaluation is critically reviewing one's performance in carrying out nursing care. Evaluation of nursing care begins with each nurse being able to give feedback to herself and to others in a supportive, non-judgemental way. It requires trust and honesty between nurses who work together.

Evaluation of the effectiveness of nursing leadership

The same self-evaluation and group evaluation exercises described earlier in this chapter can be used to evaluate how the ward leader is perceived by those with whom she works. If one wishes to use the 'best and least' exercise to evaluate nursing leadership, the group of nurses carrying out the exercise identify what they liked best and least about the ward leader's performance as the manager of nursing care: this is done in a caring, supportive and non-judgemental way. Equally, the ward leaders themselves can use a variety of techniques to identify whether their leadership style is appropriate for developing the potential of each nurse and is conducive to promoting the humanistic ideology of individualised nursing care. Examples of leadership exercises are given in Chapter 12.

Summary

This chapter began with the assumption that there are three aspects involved in evaluation: evaluation of measurable outcomes, evaluation of personal and professional growth of the nurse and evaluation of the effectiveness of the leadership style of the ward leader as the manager of nursing care. The assumption is also made that evaluating all these involves both subjective and objective evaluation strategies and that true evaluation combines all three aspects. Measuring patient outcomes is a difficult process which requires nurses to become more skilled at identifying standards of practice and performance indicators and criteria against which we can measure nursing care. We have some crude indices at our disposal, however, many of which are related to some of the points highlighted in Chapter 5 (assessment) and Chapter 6 (nursing diagnoses and planning care). But evaluation is also being flexible in nursing practice and developing the ability to admit that a chosen way of tackling a nursing problem may not necessarily meet the needs of the patient. This requires self-awareness, personal growth and professional development, which is why evaluation is about subjective measurement of personal development as well as objective measurement of patient outcomes.

References

La Monica E (1979) *The Nursing Process: a Humanistic Approach*. Menlo Park: Addison-Wesley

Section III

Chapter 8

Decision-making and Care Planning

Previous chapters make it clear that care planning involves numerous complex skills and that many of these skills are not related solely to care planning. Indeed, there is an enormous overlap between care planning skills and those involved in other aspects of a nurse's work. Decision-making skills also fall into this category of overlap because they are required for care planning as well as for a wide range of other nursing activities. Decision-making is sometimes divided into two types: managerial and ethical, although it can be argued that managerial decisions have an ethical component to them since they are about 'right' versus 'wrong' decisions. This chapter explores the following points:

- Care planning as an ethical issue
- How ethical decisions are made
- Values clarification in decisions about care planning

As in other chapters, practical exercises are offered for teachers and ward staff to allow them and other nurses to become better able to understand some of the care planning decisions they face.

Is care planning an ethical issue?

Care planning decisions have an ethical component because they involve choosing what is right or good for a particular patient. Whenever one course of nursing action is chosen in preference to another, the choice is made, knowingly or unknowingly, because it is believed to be right, good or best from a number of possible nursing care options. Many factors affect this choice, including past experiences, personal values and beliefs, other people's expectations, and professional standards and requirements. As such, any choice made about patient care is, to some extent, a moral choice because, by definition (Thompson *et al*. 1983), morality refers to standards of behaviour actually heeded or followed by individuals or groups. The words *morality, morals* and *ethics* are often mistakenly used interchangeably, and are used emotively in our society; in reality, however, there is a difference between them. *Ethics* is the study of morals (values, beliefs and behaviours): this area of study is referred to as *moral philosophy*. When we choose what care we give (because we believe it to be the right care) and the priority we will give to that care we, in effect, are making a moral choice. It is a choice which represents something believed to be good, right or best.

Here is an example: If I choose to bath a patient I do so because I believe it is right and good for him to have a bath. My reasons for determining *why* it is right and good may vary. I may feel it is right because Sister told me to do it and I believe it is right for me to do what Sister says. Equally, I may think it is right to bath this patient because the patient wants the bath and I believe that, as part of giving individualised care, a patient should have what he wants. In any event, by choosing to bath the patient, I am making a moral choice, one based on something—whatever the reason—that I believe to be right.

But what if Sister tells me to do something which I do not think is right? I may still believe that it is right to do what Sister tells me but I also believe, in this instance, that what Sister has told me to do is not right. If I do one thing, there may be some unhappy consequences for me, yet if I do another thing, there may be other consequences for me which are not comfortable. When this happens, the moral choice becomes a *moral dilemma*. Thompson *et al.* (1983) define a moral dilemma as a choice, of whatever kind, between two equally unsatisfactory alternatives.

Not all dilemmas are moral dilemmas and not all moral choices are moral dilemmas. What makes a choice a moral dilemma is that it involves a conflict between moral principles (what we believe we ought to do) and/or moral values (what we feel to be fundamentally right or good). The dilemma might be that I feel that certain values which I hold make me wish to take one course of action. But to do so may be to act against other values which I also believe to be good or right. I cannot take both actions: I must choose one or the other. The decision I must make is to choose one thing which I value over another thing which I also value.

Care planning brings many such moral dilemmas. It is worth mentioning that, as Bergman (1973) points out, moral dilemmas may exist at two levels. Firstly, there are the wider moral issues of policy which exist (such as issues of abortion, euthanasia, resuscitation). Secondly, there are the day-to-day moral issues which arise in the course of a nurse's working life. A nurse makes choices every day: some are straightforward and free from dilemma—many of them are not.

The teacher, or nurse who has a teaching role as part of her job, can help less experienced nurses come to terms with moral dilemmas. They can provide a wide variety of learning activities in the classroom or at the bedside which will enable the nurses to explore ethical dilemmas of the day-to-day kind, learn to clarify their own values and beliefs as part of the ethical decision-making process and to live comfortably with, and understand, care planning decisions which they make in the course of their work.

The ethical dilemmas which arise in everyday care planning and care giving include conflicting obligations, informed consent, patients' privacy and confidentiality, patients' rights, accountability and many more, and it is these ethical issues which will be the focus for the remainder of this chapter.

Exploring ethical decision-making

Ethical decision-making is often an unconscious process and such decisions are often made emotively rather than in a cognitive way. Because of this, nurses are often unable to understand why they feel conflict and unhappiness when they decide to take one course of action with a patient instead of another. It is also why nurses often say 'I have no choice' and feel confused and frustrated in such situations. If nurses are encouraged to think *consciously* about the process by which they make decisions of an ethical nature, they will be able to understand why they respond as they do and how they can manage the conflict. One way of helping nurses to become conscious of the process by which they might think through ethical decisions is to use an ethical decision-making model to explore critical incidents and situations which nurses have encountered. Bergman (1973) offers one such model for teaching purposes (Fig. 8.1).

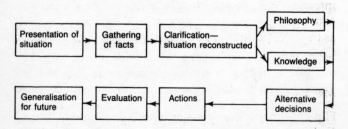

Fig. 8.1 A model for ethical decision-making (from Bergman 1973, with permission)

Bergman believes that by using the model nurses can work through ethical dilemmas of a day-to-day nature in a systematic way. By engaging in this kind of learning activity, nurses can understand their own decision-making process, deal with ethical deilemmas more satisfactorily and live more comfortably with those decisions. The model, therefore, serves as a teaching tool for both the classroom and the bedside. Students collect critical incidents—ethical situations which arise in the course of their work—and bring them to a discussion session in the classroom or at work. Incidents can be collected informally by asking students to remember them at the time of the discussion session, but they also can be collected more formally through the use of personal journals or by writing incidents down as they arise. The following exercise demonstrates how ethical dilemmas might be explored using critical incidents.

EXERCISE

This exercise should be undertaken in groups of no more than six to eight students. Prior to this exercise, students should have had the opportunity to read some background information about ethics and ethical decision-making such as those books and articles included in the references at the end of this chapter. Such background information is necessary to enable nurses to work through critical incidents intelligently and in an informed way. Prior reading and discussion should also take place about various professional ethical codes such as the UKCC, Code of Professional Conduct and the ICN Code of Conduct.

Materials

Flip-chart paper and pens or blackboard and chalk.
Copies of Bergman's ethical decision-making model (see Fig. 8.1).

Method

1   Using the technique of brainstorming, the students
    should have the opportunity to identify as many
    critical incidents as possible. A brief summary of
    the incident should be written on the blackboard or
    flip-chart by the teacher.

2   The students should then examine all the incidents
    and, as a group, put them into categories or types of
    incident. The group can label each type of category
    as they wish.

3   The groups of five to six students can now form into
    smaller groups of two or three, each of which then
    selects one of the categories or types of incident
    with which to work and later present to the others.

4   Using the ethical decision-making model (Fig. 8.1),
    the small groups of students work through one or
    more incidents from their chosen category and then
    present their work to the large group in any form
    they wish (debate, panel discussion, seminar, role
    play, etc.). The only stipulation is that the presenta-
    tion focuses on using the decision-making model to
    explore and present the incident. The groups can be
    assisted in structuring their work and their presen-
    tation by focusing on the following questions:

    (a)   What facts are known about the incident and
          what still needs to be clarified?
    (b)   What are the ethical conflicts?
    (c)   What decision was reached and what action
          was taken?
    (d)   Could alternative decisions have been taken
          which might have been more effective?
    (e)   What statements from the UKCC Code of
          Professional Conduct are relevant to this
          situation?

  Bergman's ethical decision-making model is only one
tool available for teaching students how to manage day-

to-day ethical dilemmas in care planning and care giving situations. Curtin & Flaherty (1982) have also written on ethical decision-making in nursing. They believe that it is neither helpful nor realistic to stick rigidly to only one ethical principle when confronted with an ethical dilemma. In reality, people hold many ethical principles to be important and dilemmas arise in nursing and in everyday life when different principles are in conflict with each other. Ethical dilemmas are emotive and these emotions must be explored and understood so that nurses can gain insight into emotional responses surrounding ethical dilemmas. Curtin & Flaherty also point out that it is often a difference between how we resolve a dilemma and what action we take. In other words, we resolve dilemmas by selecting which ethical principle is most important to us in a certain situation, yet we often take a different action because, despite what we believe to be right in the situation, there are often social expectations and legal requirements which influence the action we take. The ethical decision-making model put forward by Curtin & Flaherty takes into consideration many things. Their model begins by gathering the information necessary about everything and everyone involved in the dilemma. It explores the ethical principles involved in the dilemma, encourages nurses to clarify such things as rights, duties and responsibilities of the decision-maker, asks the nurse to consider options and possible consequences of each option and then assists the nurse in deciding which ethical principle outweighs the others in the particular dilemma under discussion. Their model make a distinction between deciding what is right in the situation and the subsequent action taken—which can be tempered by social expectations and legal requirements (see Fig. 8.2).

Like Bergman's model, Curtin & Flaherty ask the nurse to gather information and facts. But Curtin & Flaherty are much clearer about the extent of the background information that is required. Background information may

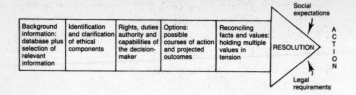

Fig. 8.2   A model for ethical decision-making (after Curtin & Flaherty 1982)

help the nurse to realise that the decision may not, in fact, be an ethical one at all. Additionally, issues which are ethical in nature may not actually be resolved by decisions which are taken by the nurse. An example of a dilemma which is ethical but which is not the nurse's decision is whether to stop treatment or not. Although there is an ethical component to this decision, it is not the nurse who makes it. The ethical decision for the nurse may well be what she does or does not do after the doctor has made the treatment decision. So, through good information gathering, the nurse can work out firstly, if the situation is an ethical one and, secondly, whose ethical dilemma it is. Curtin & Flaherty state that a situation is only an ethical one if:

- It does not belong solely to science.
- It is perplexing.
- It touches many areas of human concern.

From these three criteria it becomes clear that many care planning situations (what and how to assess, who assesses, what to do with assessment information, setting priorities, giving information, and so forth) are ethical decisions—or decisions which have an ethical component. When we seek to identify the ethical component (honesty, individual rights of people to make their own choices, justice/fairness, the duty to do good, the duty to do no harm) we seek to identify what type of ethical problem it is and whether it is in the realm of the nurse's control. Sometimes ethical dilemmas are about conflicting rights. Sometimes they are about duties and responsibilities conflicting with personal beliefs and values. Alternatively, they can be about telling the truth. Some ethical situations will, in fact, have more than one ethical component. But once these ethical components are identified by the nurse in that particular ethical dilemma, she can then be clearer about who has the authority for the decision and what effect an ethical decision taken by one health care professional will have on other health care professionals. It is only when exploring such things as duties, obligations and the degree of freedom one has in an ethical decision that all the possible options and their consequences can be identified. Some options can and will be rejected immediately: others may not.

The next step in sorting out an ethical dilemma is where the nurse reaches a stage where she understands what she values and believes to be right and choosing which principle is most important to her in this dilemma. Curtin & Flaherty use the phrase 'holding multiple values in tension' to mean that in any given ethical situation, the decision which is reached is one which is clearly understood by the nurse, which recognises that in choosing one principle over another the nurse is not rejecting other ethical principles completely and the principle chosen is one which she can defend to herself and to others.

What is appealing about the model proposed by Curtin & Flaherty is that it explicitly states that the rightness or wrongness of any ethical situation is independent of any social expectations or legal requirements and that the selection of what the nurse believes to be right in a situation must be considered separately from the legal or social expectations. It also explains how the action someone takes can be influenced by the legal requirements and social expectations and that it may differ from what the nurse believes to be right. Curtin & Flaherty's model allows the nurse, firstly, to explore the ethical nature of the situation and, secondly, to decide on an action. The exercise just described can be used in conjunction with the Curtin & Flaherty ethical decision-making model as well as Bergman's model.

Values clarification in ethical decisions

Day-to-day care planning and care giving requires nurses to select what is right or wrong nursing care. To help them to make such decisions and to be happy with the decisions that they make, nurses need to understand what they really value and how they can translate their values into their nursing practice. Steele & Harmon (1983) define a *value* as an affective disposition towards a person, object or idea. Values are individual and are formed and developed through experiences in life, from relationships with others, from the world around us and from our perceptions. A value is a stance which is taken and which is demonstrated through behaviour, feeling, attitude, imagination, knowledge and action. This is highlighted by Raths (1966) who identifies three components to a value: choosing the value, prizing it and acting on it.

We each have our values organised into some sort of hierarchical order, although we may not be aware of what it is; indeed, the order of our values may be related to specific incidents in our lives. One of the ways to help nurses make ethical decisions is to provide them with the time and opportunity to explore and clarify their own values and beliefs. It is worth mentioning that values clarification is *not* about forcing nurses to value and believe certain things. It is, however, a way by which nurses can come to know that they feel comfortable with their own values, whatever these may be. Values clarification, as a part of the ethical decision-making process, will influence the decisions nurses make about patient care. Human beings often demonstrate certain inconsistencies in their values which can cause discomfort and confusion. Values clarification is a way of resolving some of the confusion by bringing into consciousness certain parts of an individual's value system and enabling that person to examine her own values more closely. When nurses understand the things they value they can make patient care decisions in a more informed way. In an earlier part of this chapter it was stated that all care planning decisions have an ethical component to them. By exploring some of the choices made in care planning and giving, nurses have the opportunity to understand why they chose to give care when and how they did, and to identify the values which might underlie that choice. The following questions highlight the fact that even the most seemingly simple patient care decision can be concerned with values.

- Why do we make beds first thing every morning? Is the decision based on individual patient need, custom and practice or because bed-making is the most important part of nursing care in the morning?
- How do we determine that most or all baths will be given in the morning? Whose bath is more important? Who makes the decision?
- What do we do when sister/doctor/relatives tell us not to give certain information about his illness to a patient?
- What happens when a nurse is sitting and talking to a distressed patient and a more senior nurse tells the nurse to go and do something else?

These are only a few of the value-related questions or situations which happen to nurses in the course of their work. Values clarification exercises help nurses to understand why they respond to situations like these in the way that they do and what principles underlie their actions and values. The following are some values clarification exercises which can be used in the classroom or at work; further exercises are described in some of the publications to be found in the list of references at the end of this chapter.

EXERCISE 1

This exercise will help nurses to identify some of their values about nursing and enable them to compare these with other members of the group.

Materials and setting

The exercise requires a room large enough for small groups of six to eight nurses to converse without disturbing others. It does not matter how many small groups undertake it at a time. The exercise should take 45–60 minutes and requires students to answer a number of questions and discuss them in their small groups. The only materials needed are a sheet of paper with eight questions printed on it and a pen or pencil for each person.

Method

1   The teacher/facilitator hands each person a sheet containing the following statements:

   (a)   I am a nurse because ....
   (b)   As a nurse I should be ....
   (c)   As a nurse I should not be ....
   (d)   The most important thing for me to remember as a nurse is ....
   (e)   The one thing all nurses have in common is .
   (f)   I am different from other nurses in that .....
   (g)   The thing I like most about nursing is ......
   (h)   Some nurses make me angry because ......

2 Once each individual has completed the statements she should select a partner from the group with whom to discuss and share them. The facilitator can pose questions to direct their discussions, such as: How can our values influence the way we behave as nurses? In what way do our values affect our every-day nursing? How do differences and similarities in values among nurses affect the profession? Do I practise these values in my nursing?

3 If it is appropriate and the group as a whole is not too large, a general discussion can take place with the group.

EXERCISE 2

This is a game called 'HIJACK'.

Materials and setting

A room large enough for groups of four to six students to discuss the situation with minimal disturbance to other groups. There is no limit to the number of groups. The facilitator will have a passenger list for each group which contains the names of passengers on a small aircraft and a brief description of each passenger.

Suggested passenger list

A nun who is also a nurse; she is on her way to a retreat.
A pregnant woman on her way to visit her dying mother.
A 9-year-old boy who is bad-tempered, ill-behaved and has been annoying all the passengers throughout the journey.
An elderly, world-famous and distinguished Nobel-Prize-winning scientist.
A pop star, idol of millions, aged 19.
A brain surgeon on his way to an international conference.

A drug addict, aged 21, on his way to a special clinic to cure his addiction.
An MP on a fact-finding mission.

(These are just suggestions: the teacher can add or delete passengers as appropriate.)

Method

1   The teacher/facilitator announces that she has hijacked a small aircraft and has told the authorities that unless her demands are met, she will kill all of the passengers except two.

2   The students, working in groups of four to six have to decide, from the passenger list, who they would choose to save. They have 30 minutes in which to decide.

3   At the end of the time, the groups come together to discuss their choices and how they arrived at their decision.

4   During the discussion the students should be encouraged to identify what criteria they used for their decisions and what underlying values might have influenced their choices.

5   Discussion can end with the teacher encouraging students to identify nursing care situations where they might have to make difficult choices. How do they make these choices? Do their choices related to patient care reflect similar underlying values as their choices about the passengers on the aircraft?

EXERCISE 3

This is an exercise which is first carried out by individual nurses on their own, is then discussed in pairs, and is followed by a general discussion in a larger group of eight to twelve students.

Materials and setting

A room large enough to allow students to work on their own, discuss in pairs without disturbing others and then to join together for a group discussion.

Each person is given twelve small slips of paper, on each of which is written one of the following statements describing aspects of the nurse–patient relationship:

- Remaining professional with the patient
- Becoming emotionally involved with the patient
- Teaching the patient
- Disclosing myself to the patient
- Touching the patient
- Listening with empathy to the patient
- Helping to decrease a patient's anxiety
- Being honest in answering the patient's questions
- Making sure that medications and treatments are done on time
- Following doctor's orders
- Seeing that the patient does what he is told
- *One blank piece of paper for the student to write in whatever she wishes*

Process

1   Working independently, each student spends ten minutes arranging the slips of paper into her personal order of priority.
2   Each student then chooses another person with whom to discuss and share her priority list, and they explain to each other the reasons for their choices. Discussion in pairs can focus on similarities, differences, how they came to their decisions, and so on.
3   The whole group then comes together to discuss what the exercise meant to them, what they found

out about their own ways of setting priorities and how they felt about discussing their value priorities with one other person.

4   Alternatively, the students can be encouraged to write down one thing they have learned about their own values during this session and how this might influence their nursing care in the future.

These are only a small sample of the many values clarification exercises which can be used by teachers or trained nurses in teaching activities related to making eithical decisions. Values clarification is one part of the ethical decision-making process. All too often, ethical issues are seen to be those which the media highlights— abortion, euthanasia, contraception, and so forth. All stages of the care planning process contain very fundamental ethical and value-related issues. In order to enable nurses to recognise and make ethical decisions, they must be given the opportunity to clarify what they believe and value, to identify how they behave with regard to that which they value and to feel comfortable when day-to-day care planning dilemmas arise.

Summary

Values clarification activities and ethical decision-making models for teaching can be used to help nurses to explore critical incidents which arise when assessing patients and giving care. These types of activity lead to heightened awareness of what nurses do, why they do it, what alternatives are available and how they can live more comfortably with their values and the conflicts of values which arise. Care planning should aim to give care which is of the quality patients deserve. Values clarification and becoming comfortable with ethical dilemmas can help nurses to identify what high quality is and to work towards achieving it.

References

Bergman R (1973) Ethics: concepts and practice, *International Nursing Review*, **20**, 5

Curtin L & Flaherty M (1982) *Nursing Ethics: Theories and Pragmatics*. Bowie: Robert Brady

Raths L (1966) *Values and Teaching*. New York: Merrill

Steele S & Harmon V (1983) *Values Clarification in Nursing*. New York: Appleton-Century-Crofts

Thompson I, Melia K & Boyd K (1983) *Nursing Ethics*. Edinburgh: Churchill Livingstone

Additional reading

Pfeiffer J & Jones J (1974–1983) *A Handbook of Structured Experiences For Human Relations Training*, Vol I–IX. San Diego: University Associates

Simons S, Howe L & Kirschenbaum H (1972) *Values Clarification: A Handbook of Practical Strategies for Teaching*. New York: Hart

Thompson J & Thompson H (1985) *Bioethical Decision-Making for Nurses*. Norwalk: Appleton-Century-Crofts

Tschudin V (1986) *Ethics in Nursing*. London: Heinemann

Uustal D (1978) Values clarification in nursing. *American Journal of Nursing*, **78**, 12

Chapter 9

Personal Growth as a Means of Professional Growth: I Self-awareness

The preceding chapters highlight many of the complexities involved in care planning. Equally, they point out that care planning involves skills and activities which distinguish between the passive view of nursing as a list of tasks to do, and active, dynamic nursing which is skilful, thoughtful, an independent as well as interdependent activity; a questioning, seeking, ever-growing professional activity. This is the essence of professionalism. It assumes that professional growth and development occurs as a result of personal awareness, growth and development. A nurse who is aware of who she is, what she values and believes and what her strengths and weaknesses are will have the strong foundation on which to build the interpersonal skills required for humanistic care planning and care giving. Personal growth and development is divided into two parts. The first of these, self-awareness, is explored here, and in the next chapter the theme of personal growth and development continues by focusing on basic personal life skills.

What is personal growth and development?

The nursing process is a scientific, yet humanistic,

approach to caring for people. As such, it requires that nurses should have both a scientific, problem-solving approach to the problems encountered by people in need of nursing, and an individualistic, humanistic approach to people. Educational programmes in nursing have gone a long way towards fostering a scientific, problem-solving approach. What has been missing from these programmes is teaching and learning related to the humanistic and personal side of nursing. In order for people to understand and empathise with those in their care, they must learn to understand their own feelings and their own selves. Time, energy and resources must be given to enabling students to develop the self-awareness and human life skills that will allow them to explore who they are, what they feel and value and how they face and respond to human situations; to be open and honest with themselves and with others, and to trust. Peplau (1952) points out that when nurse and patient first meet, they meet as strangers: they have relatively little in common and have no reason whatsoever to trust each other or to be open and honest. It is of paramount importance that the nurse should have the ability and skill to accept the patient as he is—having no preconceived ideas and drawing no conclusions about him. A skilled nurse who is aware and responsive will assume—until it is proved otherwise—that the patient is an equal, emotionally able, sensible human being. This ability to view people as equal to oneself, and to accept people as they are, requires that the nurse accepts herself as a human being equal to others: this is the beginning of self-awareness. Teachers and trained nurses have a responsibility to help other, junior, nurses to know themselves. It is fundamental to individualised care planning that nurses know themselves first, so that they are in a good position to know their patients. Peplau also points out that, essentially, there are three ways of viewing ourselves. These are:

- 'I can identify my wants and needs, communicate them to others who respect me, and get assistance to achieve satisfaction.'
- 'I do not need to identify my wants; if I remain helpless others will give me what they think I need and I will feel safe with them; a helpless person who makes no demands will not be deserted.'
- 'I cannot count on others to give me any kind of help; they do not respect me or my abilities, but I will get what I need without help even if I have to take it.'

This may oversimplify the manner in which we view ourselves but it brings up the subject of power and powerlessness. A nurse in hospital is in a uniquely powerful position with regard to her patients. The nurse who can identify and communicate her wants and needs and can rationally seek to satisfy her own needs is in a position of personal awareness which will enable her to view her patients in the same way—that the patient is free to identify his wants and needs and to communicate them, have his needs respected and to seek assistance in satisfying them. A nurse who cannot identify and seek ways of meeting her own needs is less likely to see the need for the patient to identify his own needs. A nurse who feels helpless in the face of powerful others will often treat patients as though they are helpless in the face of her power over them. A nurse who does not feel respected by others may herself be unable to respect others and may become indifferent (even unconsciously) to the needs of her patients.

Personal awareness, growth and development will lead to nurses knowing themselves better and will enable them to begin to view themselves as Peplau described in the first of her approaches just quoted. Once a nurse is able to identify her own wants and needs, communicate these to others and seek assistance in having her needs met, she will then be more likely to allow, encourage and facilitate her patients to do the same. But to enable nurses to become aware of self and to identify their needs and seek to have them met requires time to be given in educational programmes for development of these skills. Knowing oneself and identifying one's needs is one of the most fundamental of life skills. Care planning which is humanistic and which allows the patient freedom to identify his own needs and seek to meet these needs being with a nurse who can do the same for herself first. It is from this skill of self-awareness that all other basic life skills evolve, including the following.

- Negotiation
- Assertiveness
- Making and keeping relationships
- Managing stress and conflict
- Giving and receiving praise
- Giving and receiving constructive criticism
- Coping with adversity and discomfort
- Working in groups

Many of these life skills overlap with each other but have been separated in this way in order to explain and discuss them more fully. They are all skills required for humanistic care planning and will be discused in greater depth in Chapter 10.

What do we mean by self-awareness?

Many counsellors, therapists and psychologists offer descriptions and definitions of self. One which has relevance for nursing, however, has been provided by two American nurses, La Monica and Parisi (La Monica 1985). In their model, which they call the PELLAM pentagram (see Fig. 9.1) the self is made up of five parts, each represented by the points of a star. Each part merges in the centre to form the total self—that which makes each of us totally unique as human beings. Running through each point of the star and surrounding the centre (self) is the body.

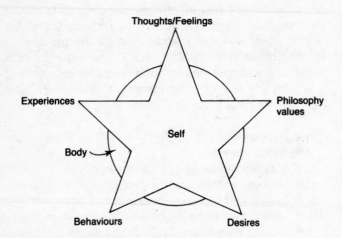

Fig. 9.1 The PELLAM pentagram (from La Monica 1985, with permission)

Fig. 9.2 shows an adaptation of the PELLAM pentagram, in which an additional element of self—the transpersonal element—is shown. This is sometimes called the spiritual dimension and is also influenced by, and influences, the five areas identified in the diagram. This model can be used by nurses and nurse teachers to give some structure and direction to all the areas of self of which nurses need to become aware. Many self-awareness and self-growth activities are available which enable nurses to develop their own awareness of themselves, and activities such as these should form an integral part of all nursing education, from basic to postbasic and continuing nurse education programmes. Any self-awareness development for nurses must include development in all areas of the pentagram: thoughts/feelings; philosophy/values; desires; behaviours; experiences.

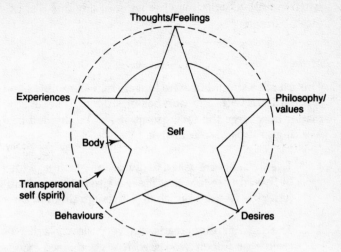

Fig. 9.2 An adaptation of the PELLAM pentagram

Developing self-awareness of thoughts/feelings

The following are a selection of activities which can form a part of a programme of self-awareness development for helping nurses to get in touch with their thoughts and feelings.

EXERCISE: THOUGHTS AND FEELINGS IN COLOUR

The purpose of this exercise is to enable students to become aware of feelings which are aroused in the course of their working day. This will help them form some composite picture of the emotional climate and attitudes in which they are working.

Materials and setting

One piece of flip-chart paper for each person and an assortment of colour pens, pencils or crayons.

A room will be needed that is large enough for several small groups to work together without any one disturbing the others.

Method

This exercise should take no longer than 45 minutes and can be done with any number of students because no matter how large the total group, it will be divided into working groups of four or five.

1   The students are asked to divide into groups of four or five and are told that the exercise is about identifying the feelings which flow through them in their work.

2   The teacher then reads out very slowly a list of twelve or fifteen words with a good-sized pause between each word. Each student listens to the words and then identifies the *major* feeling she has when she thinks of each one. She then chooses a colour pen and draws something with it on her piece of paper.

3   When the teacher has finished reading out the words and each student has drawn her series of pictures in her chosen colours, the students should spend a few minutes on their own reflecting on what they have drawn, the main characteristics of each drawing, what meanings the drawings have for them and their use of particular colours for particular drawings.

4   Students should then share their drawings with the others in their small groups, discussing similarities and differences in what they have drawn and what colours they used to describe different feelings. This should take up to ten minutes.

5   Depending on the size of the total group of students, the smaller groups of four or five can join

together to form a large whole group for a general discussion. The teacher can ask for a volunteer to show her drawings and identify such things as what colours she used most often and which emotional state is represented most often in her drawings. If time allows, other students can be invited to show their drawings and colours.

6   This exercise can be brought to an end by asking each student to identify 'One thing I have learned about myself from this exercise is . . .'

Suggested word-list for the teacher/group leader to use for this exercise

helping	professionalism	life	nursing
hospital	death	nurse	obligation
dedication	Florence Nightingale	sacrifice	uniform
community	education	doctor	patient

or any other words of her own choosing.

EXERCISE: IDENTIFYING THOUGHTS AND FEELINGS

The purpose of this exercise is to identify thoughts and feelings which are generated in nursing situations.

As with the previous exercise, total group size can be unlimited because the large group will divide into smaller groups. There can be an unlimited number of small groups.

Materials and setting

A sheet of A4 paper and a pen or a pencil for each student. The group will need a room large enough for groups of four or five to work together without disturbing others.

Method

1   The students are asked to divide into groups of four or five and are told that the purpose of the exercise is to identify thoughts and feelings which arise in certain nursing situations.

2   The students are also told that the teacher will read a short story to them but at certain places in the story she will stop and ask them to write something down using the first person—'I'—approach. The words which they write down will be related to what they think, feel or might do in the particular situation. (This will assist in separating thoughts from feelings and actions, and at the same time recognise and emphasise that thoughts, feelings and actions are related.)

3   The teacher then reads a story (see below).

4   After the story is finished and the students have written their individual responses they should share their responses with the others in their small group using discussion, drama or any other method.

5   Time should be allowed for the students, in their groups, to discuss any similarities and differences in the thoughts, feelings and actions they have identified, and how these thoughts feelings and actions related to each other in the situation.

6   The activity can end with a self-evaluation exercise such as each student identifying 'One thing I have learned from this exercise is . . .'

Suggested stories for use in this exercise

1   It is 9.00 p.m. in the accident and emergency department. The phone rang a few minutes ago and you answered it. You were told by ambulance control that an ambulance is on its way to your department from a road traffic accident. One person has died and two are seriously injured.

The ambulance arrives. Put yourself in this setting. I meet the ambulance at the entrance to the accident and emergency department. I feel . . . . I think . . . . This is what I would do . . . .

2   I have been working on my own in a four-bedded part of the ward. My four patients are fairly ill and dependent and all require a tremendous amount of my time and attention. At 10.30 a.m. I am finally able to get to my morning coffee break. As I walk out of the four-bedded bay, one of my patients rings her buzzer and calls out to me. I feel . . . . I think . . . . This is what I do . . . .

3   It is noon. The patients are having lunch. Sister has just told me to go to my lunch break. I am taking my apron off as I walk to the door of the ward when another nurse shouts 'Come quickly! Cardiac arrest!' I feel . . . . I think . . . . This is what I do . . .

Any other stories of your own choice may also be used. A variation of this exercise is to use students' actual experiences or stories.

Developing self-awareness through exploring one's philosophy/values

The second point on the star of the pentagram provides nurses with another focus for development of self-awareness. The exercises offered in Chapter 8 about values clarification are appropriate to developing self-awareness of one's value and belief systems and the reader is therefore referred to that chapter.

Developing self-awareness through exploring one's desires/wishes

Many nurses find it difficult to recognise their own wants or desires and make these known to others. Yet it is essential for nurses to be able to identify what they wish or desire in order to help their patients identify their own desires and wants. The following is an exercise to help nurses to become aware of their own wishes and desires. Further exercises can be found in the publications listed at the end of this chapter.

EXERCISE: WHAT I WANT FROM NURSING

The purpose of this exercise if to identify for each student those aspects of nursing practice which prevent it from being personally fulfilling, and to explore areas in which change is possible.

The exercise takes approximately one hour and is most effective when carried out by a group of no more than fifteen participants. Students are formed into smaller groups for part of the exercise.

Materials and setting

A large room is required where students can sit fairly comfortably. Each student needs a pen/pencil and a sheet of A4 paper.

Method

1   The teacher will read out some incomplete sentences to the students, who will then be asked to complete them.
2   In small groups of four or five, students will be asked to share their completed sentences with the others in their group. The teacher should tell the students to take note of the similarities and differences in their responses and of their individual reactions to other students' responses.
3   Still in small groups, the students should discuss their reactions, similarities and differences, how their thoughts evolved or why their responses were important to them.

4   The smaller groups can come together in a large group to tell each other what their individual groups found significant, similar or different.

5   As a large group, the similarities and differences can be explored and discussed. This often leads to a discussion about reality versus one's ideals.

6   This exercise can be closed by carrying out a 'best and least' evaluation as described in Chapter 7.

Incomplete sentences for the teacher to read out

1   If there is one thing I would change about myself as a nurse, it would be ....

2   If there is one thing I would change about my profession it would be ....

3   In five years I would like to be ....

4   Nursing is more than ....
     it is ....

5   An aspect of nursing which is missing for me is ..

6   When I was a student (or first-year) nurse my experience of being a student (or first-year) was ..

7   Now that I am qualified (or a third-year student) nursing is ....
     and I feel.....................................
     about this.

Developing self-awareness through exploring behaviours

How we behave is determined by many things: our self-concept, life experiences, how we feel at any given time, how we perceive others, and so forth. Part of developing self-awareness as a nurse is understanding how and why we behave and act. The following exercises can be used to raise awareness of how people behave in particular situations.

EXERCISE: EXPLORING BEHAVIOUR THROUGH ROLE PLAY

The purpose of this exercise is to enable nurses to examine how they perceive their own behaviour and that of others in certain situations, and to allow them to explore alternative ways of behaving in those situations.

Ideally, the group should be no larger than 20 but each role play will be carried out in very small groups. Several role plays will be happening at one time, with each group playing out either similar or different situations. Each role play will consist of three to four people.

Materials

A large room is needed, one which preferably has little or no furniture and in which people can move freely around. No other materials are required other than those which might be wanted as props for the role play, e.g. chairs, tables.

Method

1   From a list provided by the leader, each group of three or four chooses a role play situation which they wish to carry out.
2   Once the group has decided the situation, individual roles are chosen by the people in the group. Those not playing specific roles act as observers and will lead the discussion within the group after the role play. For groups who are unfamiliar with leading discussion after this sort of role play, guidelines can be given on how to be an observer, lead a discussion, and so on. (An example of such guidelines will be found at the end of this chapter: see p. 111.)
3   Each person then takes a few minutes to think about the role she will be playing, try to feel like the character she is playing and to decide what sort of attitude or behaviours she wishes to assume.

4   The role play is then carried out and should take between five and ten minutes.

5   Immediately after the role play is finished, the group should have the opportunity to discuss it. The discussion is led by the observer(s), using the guidelines.

6   The discussion ends with de-roling or de-briefing, the purpose of which is to make absolutely certain that the nurses will leave the feelings and behaviours of the role play behind them and return to being and feeling themselves. The observers can de-role the players. (Simple de-roling techniques are described in the Appendix.)

7   If time allows, the role play may be carried out a second time, either with different people playing the original roles or with the same people playing the same roles but choosing to assume entirely different attitudes.

8   The exercise can end with each student saying in turn 'One thing I have learned in this experience is . . .'

Examples of role play situations appropriate for this exercise

1   A ward meeting, handover report or case conference concerning a particular patient or problem, e.g.
     (a)   Mrs Sims in bed number 4 will not take her medication and is very uncooperative.
     (b)   The nursing team's morale is really low: no one helps anyone else and there is some direct hostility between certain nurses; the general ward atmosphere is pretty gloomy. Something has to be done.

2   Three scenes role played with the same people 'starring' in each to determine the difference in behaviour and feelings between the three situations. The three scenes are:

(a)   two nurses talking about a patient at that patient's bedside (the two nurses can agree between themselves who the patient is, what he is like and what they are talking about).

(b)   Two nurses standing in the corridor outside the ward talking about a patient.

(c)   Two nurses talking about the patient in the canteen during their lunch break. . . . .

3   A nurse is helping to feed four patients. The patients are:

(a)   Mrs Jones, who is impatient and irritable,

(b)   Mrs Smith, who is lonely and seems to want to talk,

(c)   Mrs Johnson, who is extremely worried about her condition, and

(d)   Mrs Hobson, who is apathetic, does not seem to care about anything, including her dinner.

4   A student nurse with a staff nurse and patient. The staff nurse is evaluating the care given to the patient by the student, including giving praise and constructive criticism.

The following is another exercise to allow nurses to explore their behaviours with particular emphasis on how prejudices and 'labels' affect their behaviour towards people.

EXERCISE: EXPLORING BEHAVIOURS AND LABELLING PEOPLE

Many kinds of behaviour arise out of how people perceive others. The purpose of this exercise is to explore how people behave towards others when they have, for whatever reason, 'labelled' someone as being a particular type of person.

Materials

Prior to leading this exercise, the teacher will have made

five to eight headbands to use in this exercise. Each headband is made of heavy paper or thin card and is approximately 5 × 7 inches in size, with strings attached at either end to enable it to be tied round the head. On each headband is written in clear, large, dark letters a particular role or 'label' and a brief explanation of how the other members of the group should respond to the person wearing that particular headband; for example:

Comedian: laugh at me!
Expert: ask my advice and listen to me!
Important person: defer to me!
Stupid: sneer at me!
Insignificant: ignore me!
Loser: pity me!
Boss: obey me!
Helpless: support/rescue me!

Method

1   Five to eight people will carry out this exercise and will sit on chairs in a circle in the centre of the room; any remaining people are seated outside the circle to act as observers.

2   The teacher places a headband on each student carrying out the exercise. This is done in such a way, that none of the participants can read her own headband but is able to see clearly those of everyone else.

3   The teacher then provides a topic for discussion (any topic will do) and instructs the people with the headbands to interact and discuss with each other in a way which is natural for them, e.g. to attempt to play themselves in the discussion. The participants are also asked to respond to the others in the group during the discussion by following the instructions and role written on the others' headbands. The

teacher should remind the participants not to tell the others what their headbands say, they are simply to react to them as instructed by the head-band. Only those with headbands may participate in the discussion. The others merely observe the interactions.

4   This group discussion lasts for fifteen or 20 minutes. When the discussion has ended, the teacher asks each of the participants to try to guess what is written on her headband: only then should she take it off and read what it says.

5   Both the participants and the observers should then be given the opportunity to discuss: how it felt to try to be oneself when treated by others in a way which they did not fully understand; how it felt to be constantly misinterpreted by the group, e.g. to be sneered at, ignored, laughed at; whether they found that they behaved differently in response to the way the rest of the group was treating them. The observers should tell the participants what they saw happening and any changes of behaviour that were noticeable to them.

6   To close this exercise each nurse should say 'One thing I have learned from this exercise is . . .'

Awareness of past experience

The final point in the PELLAM pentagram in Fig. 9.2 is that dimension of self which is a result of our past experiences. Part of being self-aware is understanding how past experiences make people what they are today. Being aware of the impact of past experiences on oneself enables one clearly to see how incidents from the past can affect present day choices and decisions. The following exercises will enable nurses to become more aware of the effect of past experiences upon themselves.

EXERCISE: PAST EXPERIENCES AND PRESENT NURSING
PRACTICE

The purpose of this exercise is to enable nurses to
examine some of their past experiences which may affect
their present nursing practice. The group size is unim-
portant as this exercise can take place with unlimited
numbers of small groups. The exercise takes approximately one hour.

Materials and setting

A large, comfortable room is needed where people can sit
in small groups and talk to one another. Sheets of flip-
chart paper and felt-tipped pens are needed.

Method

1   Sitting in small groups of up to six people, each
     nurse is given a piece of paper and a felt-tipped pen
     and is asked to draw a picture of the most critical
     experience she has had in her nursing practice.

2   When finished, each participant should share her
     critical experience with the rest of her group, show-
     ing her picture, explaining the experience and why
     it was critical for her, and how it affects her at
     present.

3   When everyone in the group has had a chance to
     show and explain her picture, a general discussion
     can take place which focuses on how important
     points in their careers have affected their present
     thoughts, feelings and actions as a nurse.

4   The exercise can be ended by asking each nurse to
     identify one thing she has learned from the
     exercise.

EXERCISE: LIFE EXPERIENCES WHICH INFLUENCE THE CHOICE
OF NURSING AS A CAREER

The purpose of this exercise is to enable nurses to reflect
on the life experiences which influenced their choice of
nursing as a profession.

The maximum number of participants will depend on
the size of the room available as the exercise involves the
participants lying on the floor. The exercise is carried out
in groups of three people, and takes 45 minutes.

Materials and setting

A large room is needed, preferably one that is carpeted or
with blankets which can be placed on the floor.

Method

1   Each participant is asked to lie on the floor and
    begin taking slow, deep breaths.
2   In a quiet, slow voice, the teacher gently tells the
    participants to close their eyes and close their minds
    to all thoughts and to concentrate only on their
    breathing, how their chests and abdomens move as
    they breathe, and on the floor on which they are
    lying.
3   After a few minutes' silence the teacher asks the
    participants to think back on their nursing careers
    and reflect upon certain questions. (The teacher
    then asks the following questions in a slow, gentle
    and subdued voice in order to maintain the restful,
    quiet and contemplative atmosphere. It also helps
    to have the lights dimmed and, if facilities allow, to
    have soft music in the background.)
    (a) Who was the most impressive nurse you have
         known in your life?
    (b) How old were you when you first met this
         nurse?
    (c) What was this nurse like physically?

(d) What was this nurse like as a person?

(e) What was it about this nurse which most impressed you?

(f) Why was this nurse so important to your life?

4 The questions should be asked with long pauses between each. After allowing between ten and fifteen minutes for this reflecting and reminiscence, ask the participants to get up slowly, stretch their arms and legs, and form into groups of three. Ask them to share their thoughts and reflections with their group. It may be helpful to have the questions written on the blackboard or on a piece of flip-chart paper for easier recall.

5 Following this, ask the group to identify any common or shared experiences.

6 The groups of three can join together in a total group discussion of the experience. The discussion can focus on shared or different experiences or on the effect which modelling oneself on another has in influencing social and professional development.

Some final words about self-awareness

Scheirer & Draut (1979) demonstrated that there is a strong correlation between the type of self-concept a person has and the patterns of thought and action which that person demonstrates. Although it is not clear whether it is the behaviour which affects the self-concept, or vice versa, the link between self-concepts and behaviour is there. A nurse with a positive self-concept will be secure in her values and beliefs; she will accept herself and others; she will have high self-esteem. All these characteristics are essential for the true practice of individualised care, for empathising with patients and for acting as an advocate for the patient and taking person responsibility for one's own actions. Adler *et al*. (1983) point out that people who have a positive self-concept exhibit the following characteristics:

- They are unafraid of new ways of working.
- They make friends easily.
- They trust their leaders.
- They can cooperate with others.
- They take responsibility for controlling their own behaviour.
- They try out new ideas without hesitation.
- They are creative, imaginative and have ideas of their own.
- They can share their thoughts and experiences easily.
- They are independent and can work with a minimum amount of direction.
- They are happy.

It seems apparent that many of the characteristics required to practise individualised care planning are exactly the same as those listed above. This means that a fundamental part of teaching care planning is the need to facilitate nurses' self-awareness and the building of a positive self-image.

Summary

The focus of this chapter has been the underlying theme that in order for nurses to be open and receptive to identifying and meeting the needs of patients, they must be open and receptive to their own needs through the process of becoming self-aware. Self-awareness is only one part of personal growth and development which is required by nurses if they are to relate to their patients in an individualised way. The PELLAM pentagram provides a way by which nurses can focus on all the components which make up the self. Chapter 10 continues the theme of personal growth and development in terms of how, by developing basic life skills, nurses can relate more effectively to people and better meet their needs.

Guidelines for Observing Role Play

The role of observer is fourfold:

1   To observe carefully and take note of *specific* items in the role play.
2   To allow each participant in role play to talk about their thoughts and feelings about their role play.
3   To feed back observations and lead discussion on the role play.
4   To allow role players to de-role.

This is one suggestion for how to be a useful role play observer:

1   Decide ahead of time what specifically you will be observing. The more things you try to observe the less effective will be your observation. Your choice might include:
    (a)   observing reflecting skills;
    (b)   observing types of questions used;
    (c)   observing eye contact;
    (d)   observing how well cues are taken up and used; and so forth.
    If there is more than one observer, decide in advance who will observe what.
2   Take notes (unobtrusively) about what you are observing. They need only be one or two word reminders of a point you want to remember.
3   After the role play, allow each player to talk about her thoughts, feelings and opinions about the role play. Use open questions in leading this part of the discussion. Avoid allowing the players to judge their performances as actors. Encourage each player to analyse the skills used or feelings which she recalls from the role play. Allow *each* role player to analyse her work.
4   Feed back your observations. Start with positive things and items which you thought were really helpful. Feed back how you saw the other role players respond to a particularly good question or comment. Then feed back the items which you did not feel worked quite so well in the role play. Be gentle, sensitive and constructive in your criticisms. Invite any comments on your feedback from the role players.
5   Use one of the de-roling techniques from the Appendix to end the session.

References

Adler R, Rosenthal L & Towne N (1983) *Interplay*. New York: Holt, Rhinehart & Winston

La Monica E (1985) *The Humanistic Nursing Process*. Boston: Jones & Bartlett, p 355

Peplau H (1952) *Interpersonal Relationships in Nursing*. New York: Putnam

Sheirer M & Draut, R (1979) Increasing educational achievement via self-concept change, *Review of Educational Research* (Winter), **49**, 131–50

Chapter 10

Personal Growth as a Means of Professional Growth: II Basic Life Skills

The preceding chapter focused on one aspect of personal growth—self-awareness—and the development of skills for care planning. Self-awareness and the development of self-concept is a fundamental requirement for understanding needs in others and being sensitive to these needs.

This chapter will consider other personal growth issues and the basic life skills which nurses must develop in order to build on self-awareness and to be able to relate to others in a healthy, helping way. The following life skills will be explored in this chapter:

- Assertiveness skills/negotiation
- Management of stress
- Giving and receiving praise and constructive criticism

Assertiveness skills

The ability to be assertive and to negotiate with others about one's own wishes is a fundamental and valuable skill to acquire. Many nurses have difficulty making the distinction between *assertive* behaviour and *aggressive* behaviour. Some people perceive that the only way to get what they want is to be aggressive. Others, however, find aggressiveness totally unacceptable behaviour. So what is the difference between being aggressive and being assertive?

Assertiveness involves directly telling another person what you want or would prefer in a way which is neither punishing, nor threatening, nor down-putting. Assertiveness is standing up for your rights as a human being but not at the cost of trampling on other people's rights or feelings. Assertiveness is about being gently but firmly open about one's own feelings, whether these feelings are positive or negative, and being able to express one's needs without feeling anxiety or guilt while doing so; it does not mean never being annoyed with another person but that annoyance is expressed sensitively and constructively.

Aggressiveness, on the other hand, involves expressing desires, needs or wants, feelings or opinions in a way which punishes, threatens or puts down another person. The aggressive individual aims to get her own way regardless of who she has to hurt to do so. Aggressive behaviour need not include shouting or thumping on a table: whenever one is sarcastic, manipulative or spreads gossip, one is behaving in an aggressive way. If the aggressive person wins or gets her own way, someone else is left feeling trodden upon.

A third term, which can be used to describe behaviour that is neither aggressive nor assertive, is *non-assertiveness*, also called *compliance*. Non-assertiveness involves hoping that one will get what one wishes for, but by not actively attempting to do anything to obtain it. The non-assertive person leaves it to chance that another person will guess what her needs are and then will meet them. Fig. 10.1 illustrates the differences between the three forms of behaviour.

Why be assertive as a nurse? A nurse who is able to express feelings, wants and needs in a way which is gentle, constructive, honest, open and non-threatening

If you are	Assertive	Aggressive	Non-assertive
This is how you might behave	You ask for what you want You ask directly and openly You ask appropriately You ask confidently without any real anxiety	You try to get what you want You do so in any way that works In doing so, you often cause bad feelings in others You are often manipulative and threatening and need to cajole, fight or be sarcastic	You *hope* you will get what you want You sit on your feelings You rely on others to guess what you want
This is how you would not behave	You do not violate other people's rights You do not expect people to guess what you want You do not freeze up with anxiety	You do not respect that other people have the right to have their needs met You do not seek solutions where you and the other person might both win	You do not ask for what you want You do not express your feelings You do not usually get what you want You do not upset anyone You do not get noticed

Fig. 10.1   Assertiveness—aggressiveness—non-assertiveness

is a nurse who can establish relationships which she wants, negotiate with others, take some control over things in her life and be the kind of nurse which she wishes to be. Nurses often express discomfort when they are unable to be assertive in situations which require them to be so. Assertiveness is necessary to a nurse in many work situations:

- Negotiating for the particular off-duty that she wants
- Discussing with doctors her concerns about aspects of patient treatment
- Disagreeing with a colleague, especially one in authority, about an issue
- Confronting a patient, relative, or colleague in a caring but firm manner about behaviour which is inappropriate

Why do nurses not assert themselves? Part of the answer to this question lies in cultural expectations—obedience to authority is both a part of the British and nursing ethos and is subtly rewarded in both the general and nursing culture. The ancient Christian ethic of forgiveness and turning the other cheek is still a powerful force that underpins much of our society. The culture of nursing, historically, promotes a subservient behaviour. Added to this is the fact that assertiveness is not generally perceived to be a skill which is either important or able to be learned. Many nurses do not perceive that there are alternatives to being non-assertive and some believe that being assertive is the same as being aggressive.

Hopson & Scally (1980) identify four skills which make up assertiveness:

- Knowing your rights
- Knowing what you want and saying it directly
- Asserting your own preferences
- Reviewing your own behaviour to determine if it

was the most effective way of behaving in terms of getting what you want without making the other person feel bad

Assertiveness and negotiation are similar skills. To be able to negotiate with others requires the ability to state preferences, listen to counter-arguments sensitively and calmly, and reach some form of compromise which is satisfactory to both parties and terminates with both parties feeling comfortable with a decision taken. Heron (1985), in his framework of six-category intervention analysis (see Chapter 4), identifies confronting interventions as being those which require assertive behaviour. A nurse who is skilled in using confronting interventions appropriately, will be practising assertive behaviour.

How can nurses become assertive? The beginning of assertiveness lies in becoming aware of one's own ability or lack of ability to be assertive. Raising levels of awareness about how a nurse reponds to certain situations and identifying whether behaviour is assertive, aggressive or non-assertive can occur through using activities and exercises designed to help explore past and present behaviour. Self-awareness about assertiveness helps nurses identify how they behave now in particular situations, how they would wish to behave and how they can change the way they behave.

EXERCISE

The purpose of this exercise is to help nurses to identify when assertive behaviour might be appropriate for them and to practise behaving assertively using role play. The exercise takes one hour.

Materials and setting

The role play is carried out by groups of between four and

six nurses. The room needs to be large enough to accommodate all the groups involved, or alternatively, several rooms can be used.

Method

1 Each group decides from a given list (see below) which role play situation they wish to try.
2 Roles are selected within the group. Any member who does not have a role acts as observer. (Guidelines for observers can be found at the end of Chapter 9.)
3 The teacher briefs each of the players and gives her information on what the role entails.
4 The players are given a minute or two to get into the feeling of the role, to think about the situation and how their role fits in with the situation. When each person is ready, the role play can be carried out.
5 The role play can go on for as long as the players wish and they can terminate it at any time. Following the role play, the group can discuss it using the guidelines for observers.
6 It is essential for each of the players to de-role at the end of the role play discussion (see Appendix). This can be carried out by one of the observers of the role play in each group or by the teacher.

Suggested role play situations

1 A customer who brought her television to be repaired has collected it from the repair shop. When she took it home and tried to use it, she found that it was still not working correctly. She took it back to the shop and asked for a refund or for the set to be mended properly.
   Customer Should use assertive behaviour to press for either her set to be repaired properly or her money to be refunded.

Shopkeeper Insists that he mended it perfectly satisfactorily and says he is unable to give the money back without his boss's permission, and the boss is on holiday for four weeks.

2   A nurse wants a particular weekend off to attend a friend's 21st birthday party. The ward is very short-staffed.

Nurse Should use assertive behaviour to try to get her weekend off.

Sister Insists that due to staff shortage and other people's off-duty requests, the nurse cannot have the weekend off.

3   A group of friends are going to the cinema for the evening. One of them particularly wishes to see a certain film and wants to persuade the others to agree to see the same film.

Friend 1 Uses assertive behaviour to try to persuade the others.

Friend 2 Definitely does not want to see that film.

Friend 3 Does not really care which film they see.

The teacher can add any other situations to the list of possible role play situations. Equally, the students can re-enact role play situations in which they were once involved in order to try out alternative responses.

EXERCISE

This exercise is a variation on the previous exercise. The students are asked beforehand to be prepared at the session to relate an incident in their own lives where they were not satisfied with their ability to be assertive.

Method

1   The teacher asks for a volunteer from the group to relate her experience to the rest of the group. The volunteer is encouraged to present the incident as follows:

    (a)   What did she want?

    (b)   What did she say?

    (c)   Was her response an example, in her own opinion, of assertive, aggressive or non-assertive behaviour?

    (d)   How she felt at the end of the incident?

    (e)   How could she have responded differently to bring about a different result?

2   A role play can be set up where the volunteer plays herself. The role play attempts to recreate the experience in order that she can try out alternative ways of dealing with the incident. It will be necessary for the volunteer to brief the other role players on who they are and how they are to behave.

3   After the role play, the volunteer should have the opportunity to reflect on the situation using the guidelines for discussion (see Chapter 9). She should also think how her response in role play was different from her response in the original situation.

4   Other volunteers can offer their own incidents and further role plays can be carried out. It is essential that de-roling takes place after each role play discussion (see Appendix).

Further exercises in assertiveness can be found in some of the publications listed at the end of the chapter.

Managing stress and conflict

Nursing often produces situations of stress and conflict. In order for nurses to take on the role of care planner and care giver, they must develop the resources within themselves and the skills required to manage stress and conflict in a constructive way. This may include managing their own stresses, the stresses in patients and relatives and those of their colleagues.

What is stress? Stress is a topic that is much discussed by nurses and usually has a negative connotation or is seen by them as a weakness. However, Bond (1986) makes the point that stress is not necessarily associated with bad or unpleasant happenings and, indeed, a certain amount of stress is necessary for human beings to feel stimulated, interested and excited. In nursing, there seems to be a relationship between pressure and the degree to which the resulting stimulation becomes pleasant or unpleasant. For example, a certain amount of pressure causes stimulation, and the nurse feels interested and excited about her work. This, then, is a pleasant form of pressure. Additionally, in times of little or no pressure, there can be feelings of peace and calmness which are also pleasant and restful. On the other hand, pressure which becomes too great induces overstimulation, anxiety and irritation; unpleasant feelings are commonly referred to as *stress*. Equally, and all too often unrecognised, too little pressure can make one feel unstimulated, bored and frustrated and cause a different sort of stress. No pressure at all is unstimulating. As the pressure rises, all of us reach a point where we are well-stimulated and very productive in our work, and we feel great. It is at this point that nurses feel in the best physical and mental health. Even if one comes home tired after a day's work, one tends to feel 'good tired'. Unfortunately, if the amount of pressure continues to increase and becomes too great, people start feeling too tired, unhappy and develop minor ailments of one sort or another. If pressure increases further and the nurse does not have the personal skills to manage it well, ailments become more frequent, depression can occur and a state now referred to as 'burnout' can result where the nurse no longer functions productively, begins to hate her work and no longer cares about herself and others.

Stress in nurses One major problem which has its roots

in the historical development of nursing is that stress is perceived by many nurses to be a sign of weakness and of not coping, so it often goes unacknowledged, unrecognised and, consequently, unmanaged. Nursing research by Clark (1975), Redfern (1981) and others all show that stress in nurses is common and is a cause of sickness, absenteeism and wastage in nursing. The constructive management of stress is thus an important personal skill for all nurses to develop.

Bond points out that the transition from a healthy, stimulating, productive amount of pressure to that which is too great and causes stress and illness can be a gradual one and therefore difficult to recognise. This is one reason why it is particularly good for nurses to be able to explore the causes of their own stress, how stress affects their behaviour and feelings and how to manage their own stress. Stress in nurses has negative physical effects, effects on emotions, on feelings and on behaviour (Bond 1986).

Nurses who recognise stress in themselves, are aware of how it is caused and manage it well, will more likely be able to recognise it and its causes in others and help them to manage their stress. Assessing patients as a part of the care planning process includes being able to identify stress in patients and plan appropriate ways of helping them to manage it.

Nurse teaching programmes should include strategies for understanding what stress is, recognising it in oneself and others, identifying ways in which we manage stress already (although we may not realise that we are doing so) and identifying other ways in which to manage our own stress and that of others.

Cox (1978) points out that stress can be examined in six ways:

- How it makes one feel.
- How it makes one behave.
- How it affects the way one thinks.

- What happens to one's body.
- What happens to one's health.
- How it affects one's work.

In exploring stress, nurses can begin by identifying their own reactions to it. The following exercise may help.

EXERCISE

This is a small group exercise best done in groups of between three and five nurses, the purpose of which is to identify ways in which the individuals in the group react to stress.

Materials

Each group needs a sheet of flip-chart paper and a felt-tipped pen.

Method

1   One member of the group acts as a scribe.
2   The scribe should divide the sheet of paper into six sections corresponding to Cox's list above, namely:
    (a)   How stress makes me feel.
    (b)   How stress makes me behave.
    (c)   How stress affects the way I think.
    (d)   How stress affects my body.
    (e)   How stress affects my health.
    (f)   How stress affects my work.
3   The group beings the exercise by brainstorming. This means that everyone, as she thinks of something, shares her reactions or responses to stress and as each person contributes, the scribe writes it in the appropriate section of the sheet of paper. This part of the exercise should take approximately 15 minutes. At the end each group should have a comprehensive list of everyone's responses

to their own stress. There need not be agreement from everyone on all items; as long as one person identifies it as a response to stress, then it is included on the list.

4   At the end of this brainstorming session, each group should display their list on the wall so that all the groups' lists are visible to everyone. Everyone in all the groups should spend a few minutes observing and thinking about all the lists, taking particular note of:
    (a)   similarities,
    (b)   differences,
    (c)   what points on various lists particularly 'ring bells' for them.

5   Discussion can take place either in pairs or groups, during which time people can share their thoughts and observations.

6   A good way to end this exercise is for all the participants to say 'One thing I have learned about myself from this exercise is . . .'

This exercise can form a good introductory session to exploring personal responses to stress and can be followed by other sesssions on causes of stress. An example of such an exercise comes from Bond (1986) and is used with permission.

EXERCISE

The purpose of this exercise is to allow nurses the opporunity to identify the things that cause them stress. This exercise is best carried out in groups of between three and five nurses.

Materials

Each group should have a sheet of flip-chart paper and a felt-tipped pen.

Method

1   One person acts as scribe.
2   The scribe should divide the sheet of paper into three sections which are labelled as follows:
     (a) Causes of stress from other people.
     (b) Causes of stress from within myself.
     (c) Causes of stress from the world at large.
3   Using the technique of brainstorming (see previous exercise) the members of the group identify things which cause stress in themselves under any of the three headings. This should take approximately fifteen minutes.
4   At the end of the brainstorming session, the compiled lists should be displayed on the wall as described in the previous exercise and discussion can follow in the same way.

Identifying how nurses respond to stress and what causes stress is a good way of raising awareness about stress. Exercises like those just described should, however, be followed by other exercises to enable nurses to identify ways of managing stress in themselves and others and offering, wherever possible, additional strategies for doing this.

Many nurses are unaware that they already employ effective strategies for stress reduction in their lives. It is helpful to offer nurses exercises through which they can become aware of those techniques which they already use to manage stress so that they may consciously use them both to prevent and manage stress in the future.

EXERCISE (from Bond (1986), and used with permission)

The purpose of this exercise is to enable nurses to become aware of the many resources they already employ to prevent and manage stress. It allows them to identify and celebrate the constructive methods that they use to deal with stress, and by sharing these, they may be offering suggestions to others in the group on how to manage and prevent stress.

Materials

Four sheets of flip-chart paper and a felt-tipped pen.

Method

1   The teacher acts as scribe and displays the four blank sheets of paper in a row on the wall.
2   Each piece of paper has a heading as follows:
    (a)   Managing/preventing stress by using physical of mental distraction.
    (b)   Managing/preventing stress by self-nurturing.
    (c)   Managing/preventing stress by confronting the situation.
    (d)   Managing/preventing stress by emotional release/expression.
3   The teacher asks the group as a whole to call out those ways they know of, themselves use, or have heard about which fit any of the four categories on the sheets of paper. As each suggestion is offered, it is recorded on the appropriate sheet by the teacher.

The suggestions offered may include the following:

Physical/mental distraction   Sport, hobbies, taking a walk, yoga, running, massage, reading, listening to music, housework, meditation, gardening, and many others.

Self-nurturing   Long hot bath, prayer, relaxation techniques, get away from it all, go on holiday, yoga, meditation, listen to music, massage, and many others.

Confronting the situation   Get advice on how to deal with a problem, fantasy (imagining ways in which you would really like to deal with the situation), asserting your needs/wants, learning how to say no, direct confrontation with someone, changing your lifestyle (confronting yourself), and many others.

Emotional expression 'Get it off my chest by talking', writing a diary/journal, running, crying, joining a support group, bashing a cushion, and many others.

It is important to make the point that some stress reduction activities will fall into more than one category. Remember, too, that these suggestions are only examples of what might be offered by a group. Each group of nurses may identify different things and some suggestions will be offered which are not mentioned here.

4   The resulting four lists of suggested ways of managing stress will form the content for any future work the group may undertake in learning new techniques for the management of stress. Some stress reduction techniques like yoga, massage, meditation or relaxation techniques may be unfamiliar to many in the group. Others in the group who have expertise and interest in any of these areas should be encouraged to show the rest of the group some of the basic tecniques.

One of the problems which arise from this exercise is that some of the stress reduction techniques offered require people with particular skill in their performance to teach others. Anyone interested in helping nurses to manage stress may need to seek advice and help in order to learn some of the stress reduction techniques before attempting to teach them to others.

Giving and receiving praise and constructive criticism

Praise and constructive criticism are important for all people. Nurses and patients alike need to be given praise as well as constructive criticism. Appropriate use of the two enables individuals to learn more about themselves and about the effect their behaviour might have on others, and certain guidelines should be followed to ensure that praise and cosntructive criticism are useful.

Constructive criticism and praise, when given skilfully, make the person feel good about himself even if something negative has been said. Destructive feedback given in a hurtful, unskilled way leaves the other person feeling bad, angry or rejected with nothing upon which to build or improve or change in the future.

Nurses often appear unable to give and receive both praise and constructive criticism, or have some difficulty in doing so: the following are suggestions why this may be so.

Why do we find it hard to give praise?

- We are too busy and forget to praise others.
- We are more alert to people's weaknesses than to their strengths.
- We are embarrassed.
- We think the other person might become 'bigheaded'.
- No one has ever praised us, so why should we praise anyone else?

Praise, however, makes people aware of their own strengths and motivates them to carry on, to improve, to start praising others and to feel good about themselves.

Why do we find it hard to criticise constructively?

- We think that people will be upset by it so we do not bother to criticise them at all.
- We have only been criticised destructively ourselves so we do not know how to offer constructive criticism to others.

- We think that people who need criticising need to be told off.
- The other person might misinterpret, misunderstand or mistrust what we say.

Hopson & Scally (1982) offer a list of skills of giving praise and constructive criticism. These include the following:

- Be clear in your own mind about what you want to say. Practise it with another person beforehand, if necessary.
- When assessing or evaluating someone else's work, begin with positive things first.
- Be specific—avoid generalisations. Rather than saying 'You were great' or 'You were terrible', pinpoint as exactly as possible what the person did which was 'great' or 'terrible'.
- When giving praise or criticism, praise or criticise the *behaviour* rather than the person.
- Select areas of priority: do not save up criticisms from the past three weeks and throw them all at the person at one time.
- When criticising, make sure that it is something which the person is in a position to change.
- Offer alternatives, but preface suggestions by first asking the person, 'Can I make a suggestion . . .?' Heron (1985) in discussing prescriptive interventions (see Chapter 4) makes the point that although nurses often given advice, a truly valid piece of advice is one which seeks permission from the other person for the advice to be given. This allows the person the choice to accept or reject the suggestion.
- Own the praise and criticism you are giving: what this means is that rather than saying 'You are . . .' say, instead, 'I feel you are . . .'
- When you give praise or criticism, the way it is done is a reflection of yourself. Think about what

your way of praising or criticising is saying about you.
- Praise or criticism is most effective if it happens as soon as possible after the event.

A nurse who gives praise or constructive criticism in a way which helps another person to grow is one who is creating an environment for all the other care planning skills.

What about receiving praise and criticism? Nurses can help themselves to manage well the praise and constructive criticism they receive by considering the following:

- Listen to the praise or criticism and think about it rather than immediately rejecting, accepting or arguing about it.
- Clarify what has been said. Heron (1985), when describing catalytic interventions (see Chapter 4), identifies the skill of 'checking for understanding'. This skill is one way nurses have of clarifying what has been said.
- When receiving praise, accept it for what it is. Do not deny it or attempt to make it any less than it is.
- Check it out with others rather than rely only on the source from which it came. This is especially important with criticism.
- If you receive neither praise nor criticism in your work or relationships, ask for it, e.g. 'Sister, how do you feel I am getting on?'
- Decide what, if anything, you yourself wish to do with the praise or criticism.

The following is one of a number of simple positive/negative feedback exercises which may be helpful for nurses to practise giving and receiving praise and criticism.

EXERCISE

This is called 'Gifts of Happiness' (Pfeiffer & Jones, 1974) and is suitable for giving nurses experience in positive feedback and praise. The exercise, which takes about 45 minutes, requires a group of students who have had some experience of working together as a group and is best undertaken with a group of no more than twelve people.

Materials

Each nurse will need small slips of paper, one slip for every person in the group, and a pen or pencil.

Method

1   The teacher introduces the activity as follows:
    'Sometimes we become so entangled in the every-day business of life that it is easy to forget how good it feels to receive praise or positive feedback. It is also true that small gifts are often more special than large ones. In the following experience we will all be giving a small gift of happiness to each person in the group.'
2   The teacher then invites each student to write on the slips of paper a message to every other member of the group. The messages are intended to make each person feel good about herself.
    Note: the teacher may wish to give additional instructions, such as:
    (a)   Try to be specific about your message.
    (b)   Write a *special* message for each person.
    (c)   Write something for *every* member of the group.
    (d)   Try to tell each person in your message what you perceive to be a specific strength, success or attribute.

(e) Personalise the message by including the person's name in the message.

3 The teacher should encourage the group members to sign their names to the messages, but this is optional.

4 When all have finished writing a message for everyone else, they should fold their slips of paper in half and distribute them to the relevant individuals.

5 All should then read their gifts (messages). Discussion can follow in a variety of ways, e.g.

(a) Each participant can share one gift which was most meaningful with the rest of the group.

(b) Each participant can share how she felt doing this exercise.

Summary

The nursing process and care planning require sensitive and sophisticated interpersonal skills development, as earlier chapters have demonstrated. Chapters 9 and 10 have argued that in order for nurses to develop the interpersonal skills required for care planning, they must first explore and develop their own personal skills. In many ways, these two chapters should have come at the beginning of this book since much of what is discussed in Chapters 9 and 10 is essential to the skills required for care planning. But in reality, personal and interpersonal skills development are concurrent activities because through structured exercises and activities people learn more about themselves at the same time as they learn about relating to each other. The important issue which is raised in these chapters and, indeed, throughout the book, is that teachers, clinical nurses and managers have a responsibility to help other nurses to develop, both personally and interpersonally. In order to give individualised care and to be sensitive to the individual needs of others, nurses must be confident and feel comfortable with themselves. The skills highlighted in Chapters 9 and 10—those relating to personal awareness and development—enable nurses to develop confidence and comfortableness with themselves. From this confidence in oneself comes the ability to relate to others.

References

Bond M (1986) *Stress and Self-Awareness: A Guide for Nurses*. London: Heinemann

Clark J (1975) *Time Out? A Study in Absenteeism Among Nurses*. London: Royal College of Nursing

Cox T (1978) *Stress*. London: Macmillan

Heron J (1985) *Six Category Intervention Analysis*, second edition. Guildford: University of Surrey Department of Educational Studies

Hopson B & Scally M (1980) *Lifeskills Teaching Programme No. 1*. Leeds: Lifeskills Associates

Hopson B & Scally M (1982) *Lifeskills Teaching Programme No. 2*. Leeds: Lifeskills Associates

Redfern S (1981) *Hospital Sisters*. London: Royal College of Nursing

Section IV

Chapter 11

A Skills Workshop Programme for The Introductory Course of an RGN Programme

Terry Maunder and Janice Scott

Experiential learning occurs when a learner or participant engages in a particular activity, reflects upon it, draws useful insights from it, and subsequently puts these insights into practical use. Peters (1967) argues that 'to be educated is not have have arrived at a destination, it is to travel with a different view'. Experiential learning activities enable learners to examine their feelings and attitudes and allow individuals not only to understand how they are behaving in the activity but also how others in the activity also behave and what effect this behaviour has on them (Martin & Chai 1985). These techniques have evolved from student-centred philosophies of education and humanistic psychology which take the point of view that all human beings are motivated to grow and learn and have the urge to expand, extend, become autonomous, develop and mature (Rogers 1961). The nursing process is concerned with encouraging these same activities in patients and it is therefore appropriate that the way nurses learn should be congruent with this thinking.

Unlike more didactic teaching where the teacher 'talks at' the student, experiential learning takes as its starting point the student's own feelings and behaviour rather

137

than the subject matter, textbook or lesson. Insight drawn from experiential learning activities will indirectly improve patient care and the nursing process by facilitating the development of the interpersonal skills of nurses and by fostering self-awareness. Nurse teachers and clinical nurses involved in teaching nurses in a programme leading to registration as a general nurse can play a part in the development of these skills.

How we approached this teaching

As teachers in a basic RGN programme we initiated a series of experiential sessions with a group of student nurses in their introductory course. There were 27 student nurses in this group and each session involved the two facilitators working with half the group at a time. The teachers took it in turn to facilitate each session and each session was evaluated by co-supervision so that both teachers had the opportunity to explore their feelings and thoughts about the processes which had occurred during the session. Co-supervision, in this instance, is an analysis or re-construction of the lesson whereby the teacher can, through discussion, re-experience the lesson and draw insight to improve future teaching. It is, if you like, an experiential process itself.

One strand of the skills programme involved five lessons of communication, the aims of which were to develop greater insight into the skills required for the promotion of effective communication. They were seen as a basis on which to build interpersonal and personal skills and the aims were broad enough to encompass communication in all areas of interpersonal relationships: peer/peer, patient/nurse, nurse/teacher, and so forth. Planning involved moving from the concept of communication, its importance in a caring relationship through to experience in role play (e.g., nurse/patient interviews on admission). Research was used to reinforce the point that, as a profession, nurses do not communicate effectively to the extent that 'the majority of communications students used with patients (85%) were inhibitory to the communication process' (Gott 1984). An experiential focus was maintained because 'maturity, responsibility, insight and the ability to cope with stress in oneself and others cannot be learned by just watching and listening' (Briggs 1974). It was stressed that communication is an integral part of the nursing process and attention was drawn to the fact that in wards where talking is frowned upon, patients 'suffer a slower rate of recovery, greater pain and increased anxiety' (McLeod-Clark & Bridge 1981).

The second strand, following theoretical sessions on the sick role and the sociology of institutions, involved the students in an exercise which explored the sociology of families and its relevance to the students with regard to the everyday people with whom they would be entering into a helping relationship. This exercise involved role play which provided feeling experiences to enable the student to understand family situations, roles, relationships and attitudes of other people. As well as role play, a technique called 'sculpting' was carried out. Sculpting is a way of encouraging physical demonstration of an interactional situation (Tomlinson *et al*. 1984). The aim of this role play and sculpting session was to foster a holistic approach to patient care by enabling students to explore communication, conflict, power and roles within families and thereby appreciate that the people they nurse may belong to either destructive or supportive families.

The final strand involved the use of games to explore the concept of trust. The aim of this was to relate the experience of the games to the trust required in a nurse/patient relationship. A second aim was to foster the experience of trust within their own peer group.

How we arrived at our programme

We took the opportunity to have lengthy discussion and

exploration before we implemented our programme in order to ensure that we ourselves felt adequately prepared. The following is the plan for each lesson which we decided upon in our pre-course planning.

Lesson 1

This was a role play and sculpting exercise whereby role players were first briefed about the family situation by other students who played the part of presenters. This means that the presenters determined what the situation would entail and what type of parts the role players would assume within the family scene. The situation chosen for the role play was a family sitting around the breakfast table as the long-awaited 'O' level results arrived through the letterbox. The family included mother, father, boyfriend, daughter and grandmother. The role play was carried out several times in several different ways depending on the briefing of the players by the presenters. Other students in the class played the part of observers, whose role it was to sculpt the feelings and relationships as they perceived them after the role play. This exercise can be represented briefly in Fig. 11.1.

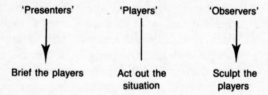

Fig. 11.1 Representation of the role play/sculpting activity

The 'presenters' briefed the 'players' separately on how they should behave during the role play. The 'observers' were asked to pay particular attention to conflict, power, communication patterns and roles (e.g. nurturing, supporting, etc.) within the interaction. Previous experience in facilitating this lesson has taught that it is also useful to invite the 'presenters' to sculpt their 'players' after the role play, if they so wish, and to permit students to tell the 'players' which pose or sculpted position to adopt rather than to perform the sculpture in silence. This appears to be less threatening to students.

Following the role play the 'observers' reported that they saw and felt the following: conflict, subservience, comfort, aggression, betrayal, shock, stress, unhappiness, arrogance, indignation, frustration, anger, sadness, bitterness, interference.

The 'players' reported that they felt: disappointment, sympathy, isolation, concern, rebellious, shocked, protective, angry, irritated, embarrassed, confused, betrayal, powerlessness, would someone hit me?

The 'observers' then sculpted the 'players'. This means that they asked them to assume statue-like positions which represented what the 'observers' saw happening in the role play and what they wanted to happen.

Example 1   One group of observers sculpted the family as follows:

Father—sitting on a chair on top of the dining table (the observers indicated that this is how they represented his dominant manner).

Mother—standing some distance away with her head bowed.

Daughter—with her arm around her boyfriend, looking at her mother.

Boyfriend—with his arm around girlfriend making obscene gestures at father.

This is an example of how observers sculpted what they saw happening in the role play with regard to power, communication within a family and roles.

The observers then sculpted the family groups as they would have liked them to be—as demonstrated in Example 2.

Example 2 All four members of the family were sculpted sitting around in a circle on four chairs and holding hands.

The students playing the parts of mother, father, daughter and boyfriend for the role play and sculpting were invited to say how these moves felt. All those involved were then de-briefed (see Appendix) by writing a statement on a piece of paper, screwing the paper up into a tight ball, throwing it onto the floor with some force and at the same time, shouting out their real names. The statement they were asked to write on the paper was:

> 'The feelings I had and saw expressed belonged to role play.'

Discussion then ensued on how this role play and sculpture could relate to patients and how what they learned from the exercise would influence their behaviour in the clinical area. The session was evaluated using the 'most and least' method in which the students write on a piece of paper what they liked most about the session and what they liked least. This type of evaluation provides feedback to the facilitators and some of the comments are included later in the chapter.

Lesson 2

This involved the use of games and structured exercises to explore the concept of trust in the nurse–patient relationship. The specific exercises used were:

- Blindfold walk
- Wall crash
- Backward fall and catch

Before embarking on these trust exercises, exercises were done with the group to energise the students and reduce inhibitions. The energiser exercise chosen was called Group Yell (Brandes & Phillips 1978). Following the three trust exercises the students evaluated their own learning during the exercises by participating in a round of statements beginning with the phrase 'One thing I discovered from doing these trust exercises was . . .' Comments included:

'If you trust someone once, you can trust him again.'
'You have to work hard at making people trust you.'

Discussion followed which focused on the development of trust between nurse and patient, embracing such concepts as acceptance, genuineness and empathy.

Lesson 3

This involved starting with a warm-up exercise and then proceeding to a group discussion to establish what was meant by the phrase 'communication between individuals' using the brainstorming technique. This is a group discussion technique whereby each member of the group is encouraged to give his/her own opinion because the rule is that no judgement is passed on anyone's contribution. All contributions to the brainstorming discussion are accepted non-judgementally. As well as exploring what is meant by communication between individuals, barriers to communication were also discussed using the insights and experiences which the students themselves had gained during their own life experiences. Research by Gott (1984), Briggs (1974) and McLeod-Clark & Bridge (1981) was cited to reinforce the point that research has been carried out which indicated that nurses do not communicate effectively, and that in order to build on the skills which students bring with them into nursing, it is important to use the classroom environment as a practice area for communication skills development.

Lesson 4

This session began with a discussion of effective communication which members of the class either had witnessed or in which they had been personally involved. This led into the exploration of the concept of 'active listening' and 'free attention', using eye contact exercises, for example, to highlight the difficulties involved when employing such strategies to enhance communication between nurse and patient. These skills are essential in being able to assess and plan nursing care and form the kind of therapeutic nurse–patient relationship required to practise patient-centred, individualised care.

Lesson 5

This lesson focused on questioning techniques and began with an initial discussion about the types of questions students had witnessed during their visits to clinical areas. Specific questions heard were collated and included the following examples:

> 'Are you in pain?'
> 'Did you sleep well?'
> 'Are you warm enough?'
> 'What's bothering you?'
> 'Are you comfortable?'
> 'Do you want a cup of tea?'

From the collated list of questions, only 10% were open-ended questions. Discussion within the group explored both 'open' and 'closed' questions. The question game described previously in Chapter 5 was used. Many students commented on how difficult it was for them to formulate open questions and discussion followed about the importance of developing the ability to use such questions. This session was seen by the students to be particularly effective.

Lesson 6

This was an optional session which involved the use of role play. The authors had learned from their own previous experiences that such lessons needed to be made optional in the timetable to avoid the likelihood of peer pressure. The lesson began with a discussion which drew on the students' experiences of interviewing patients as part of their initial visits to the clinical area. The role play began with one of the facilitators playing the role of a ward nurse admitting a patient in an 'inappropriate' manner, with a volunteer playing the part of the patient. The second facilitator dealt with feedback from the observers. The students then divided into pairs and role played an admission interview between a nurse and a patient. De-briefing was carried out and a discussion ensued related to the difficulties encountered so that students were able to give support and advice to each other in the discussion by focusing on the thoughts, feelings and intuitions which they had experienced as part of the role play process.

Lesson 7

This, the final lesson of the introductory course, was devoted to exploring students' feelings about their first ward experience. Each student was asked to write a statement or question about a possible patient situation which was worrying her, e.g. 'How do I handle a patient who has given up on life?' The statement and questions were placed in a box from which each student in turn was asked to withdraw one piece of paper and read the message on it. Each statement was discussed by the group. Conducting a session in such a way enables the students to feel comfortable when identifying something which is worrying them and yet frees them from having to admit openly what their fears or anxieties are. At the end of the lesson, the students were invited to play a game called 'The Gifts of Happiness' (Pfeiffer & Jones 1974) as a way of providing support and positive feedback. The students were advised to keep their 'gifts' as a resource in a time of stress.

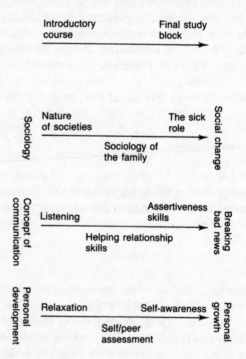

Fig. 11.2 A suggested framework for teaching social, personal and interpersonal skills in a three-year RGN programme. NB: The areas identified are a *few* examples of topics to be addressed. In reality, the process would be more complicated than indicated

Future plans

The facilitators plan to continue skills workshops throughout the three-year training, drawing upon their skills in communication, sociology and humanistic psychology. They will continue to use a variety of experiential teaching strategies such as role play, sculpting, relaxation, fantasy/imagery. Fig. 11.2 is a suggested progression for this type of interpersonal skills training. The areas identified are only a few examples of the topics to be addressed and the facilitators are aware that the process is more complex than indicated. In addition, a support group for the students has been initiated to provide a forum for discussion and for the additional development of personal and interpersonal skills.

How do the students feel about the programme?

The following comments are drawn from a wide range of evaluative comments which the students wrote during the various 'most and least' evaluation sessions at the end of lessons.

> 'I have preferred the sessions where we do role play because I have been able to actually face my feelings and to understand the feelings of patients in that situation.'
> 'The sessions were interesting because everyone was involved. I enjoy active participation because I learn more and what we do learn is from our own experience. I feel I have learnt a lot.'
> 'I've found that actually being put into a situation, i.e. role play, has given me a deeper insight into human behaviour. I think sometimes there is too much superficiality and it's really good that we are encouraged to build relationships.'
> 'The role play session was not particularly enjoyable because I found it hard to relax into it. However, the discussion and comments that arose were really good.'
> 'I liked leading 'blind' people best because I thought this exercise helped us to understand the true meaning of trust. Thank you.'

'Having teachers obviously interested in the work at hand helps everyone to learn and encourages students a great deal.'

'It's really good to know that you care enough to plan these sessions. You try hard to make the lessons thought provoking and it makes us try harder too.'

How do the facilitators feel about the programme?

These lessons were enjoyable and exciting for us, but also tiring. Time is needed afterwards for de-briefing and co-supervision. It is recommended that teachers using experiential techniques have free periods in the timetable immediately following such sessions to allow for de-briefing. Experience has also taught that such lessons need to be facilitated in pairs to maximise co-supervision and to reduce stress.

Summary

Experiential techniques have a useful role in nurse education, particularly in respect of helping students focus on their feelings and developing the wide range of personal and interpersonal skills required to give holistic care. One final recommendation is that teachers should on no account use techniques which they have not directly experienced themselves. This requires that teachers must seek ways of learning and experiencing these teaching methods. The authors also consulted a variety of critiques of experiential learning (e.g. Burnard 1984) prior to commencing the programme described in this chapter. It also is necessary to consider techniques which could be employed to cope with any strong feelings which students might experience and wish to discuss after these sessions. One such technique is for the facilitators to stay behind in the classroom after a session in order to allow students the opportunity to seek, if they wish, both physical and psychological support.

The experiences of teaching in this way are both challenging and rewarding to student and teacher and provide the opportunity to develop the personal and interpersonal skills required to give holistic nursing care.

References

Brandes D & Phillips H (1978) *The Gamester's Handbook*. London: Hutchinson

Briggs A (chairman) (1974) *Report of the Committee on Nursing*. London: HMSO

Burnard P (1982) Through experience and from experience. *Nursing Mirror*, **156** (9), 29–34

Burnard P (1984) All that glistens. *Nursing Mirror*, **160** (20), 32–3

Gott M (1984) *Learning Nursing*. London: Royal College of Nursing

Martin P & Chai T (1985) What's in a name? *Nursing Times*, **81** (20), 59–60

McLeod-Clark J & Bridge W (ed) (1981) *Communication in Nursing Care*. Chichester: John Wiley & Sons

Peters R S (1967) *The Concept of Education*. London: Routledge and Kegan Paul

Pfeiffer J & Jones J (1974) *A Handbook of Structured Learning Experiences for Human Relations Training*, Vol IV. San Diego: University Associates

Rogers C (1961) *On Becoming a Person*. London: Constable

Tomlinson A *et al.* (1984) Role play—learning to relate. *Nursing Times*, **80** (38), 48–51

Chapter 12

A Nursing Process Workshop for Nursing Officers

Sylvia P. Docking

Introduction

When the City and Hackney Health District began to
implement the nursing process, a number of in-service
educational programmes and workshops were organised
for all grades of nursing staff which would enable them to
prepare themselves for this change in their nursing practice. One such programme was begun for nursing officers
and it was felt that their needs with regard to this new
care planning and care giving system were slightly different from those of the direct care givers. The role which
the nursing officers would have to play in implementing
this change required a different sort of in-service educational programme.

The type of learning and skills development required of
nursing officers for implementing the nursing process
was such that a variety of teaching methods and
approaches were selected for their programme including
several experiential activities. This chapter will describe
the workshop programme designed for nursing officers
and will focus primarily on the teaching methods
employed rather than on details of the content of the
programme.

The Nursing Officers' Workshop

The workshop was based on the assumption that nursing officers required an understanding both of the nursing process and of the process of change, and that an integral part of their role in relation to the nursing process was to act as facilitators of change. It was hoped that, through the workshop activities, each individual nursing officer would be enabled to meet the demands of change and lead their staff through this radical change of approach to their nursing.

The workshop was a three-day programme with a two-week interval between workshop days. The aims of the workshop were:

- To enable the nursing officers to act as facilitators of change in the health district's nursing process project.
- To deepen the nursing officers' understanding of the nursing process and the process of change.
- To develop an awareness of the nursing officers' individual strengths and weaknesses about the nursing process and the management of change.
- To identify and explore specific skills required by nursing officers to help their nurses implement the nursing process.

Day 1

The first day of the workshop began with a brief introduction to the three-day programme. This introduction was led by two facilitators and was followed by a 'warm-up' exercise designed to enable participants to feel more comfortable working with each other.

WARM-UP EXERCISE

This exercise is sometimes referred to as 'Getting to Know You'.

Materials

None required except for a room large enough for all participants to sit and talk quietly in pairs and yet not disturb any other pair with their conversation.

Method

1   The participants pair off, preferably with someone they do not know very well.
2   Each pair finds themselves some space in the room to sit comfortably next to one another without disturbing others.
3   In their pairs, the participants should spend a few minutes talking and listening to each other, exchanging information about each other such as: names, outline of their role as they see it, previous experience of any other small group workshops they have attended, their expectations of this three-day nursing process workshop. The last point is encouraged through asking each person to consider these questions:
    (a)   What do I want/expect from the workshop?
    (b)   How do I feel about it right now?

Following this warm-up exercise, the subject of innovation and change was introduced using lecturette and discussion. The aim of this session was to foster awareness of their own attitudes to change, to increase their receptivity to change and to foster creativity. The facilitators began with a brief introduction to innovation and change and outlined some of the conditions which are conducive to change, the characteristics of a change agent and some of the problems and difficulties encountered when trying to make change. The participants were given the opportunity to explore the concept and problems of change in small groups. It was through these small group discussion sessions that individual and group concerns about change were identified and these concerns became the focus of much of the remainder of the workshop days. By the end of the morning, through group discussion and negotiation, the participants had identified a list of what they wished to learn and explore further during the workshop.

The participants then began to examine some of these issues. Following a discussion on the values and beliefs underlying individualised care planning and the nursing process, participants expressed the need to work on one of the concerns which seem common to all of them—the fact that none of them had ever taken a nursing history themselves nor had any of them written a care plan. The nursing officers felt de-skilled because their ward sisters, staff nurses and even the most junior of students were more experienced in doing this than they. They felt that the workshop setting might be a relatively safe place for them to try these things out. The rest of the afternoon of day 1 of the workshop centred on giving each of the participants an opportunity to take a nursing history from a patient. Each nursing officer went up to one of the wards—other than a ward on his/her own unit—and took a history from a patient. When they had finished interviewing their patient, the nursing officers returned to the classroom and shared their thoughts and feelings about the nursing histories they had taken. They discussed things which made them anxious about taking the history, questions or areas of the nursing history with which they felt comfortable, and shared their histories with each other. This session allowed the nursing officers to reflect back on the experience of taking a history to enable them to plan future action or identify areas in which they would like further practice and development.

Day 1 of the workshop ended with a brief evaluation exercise.

EXERCISE TO CLOSE DAY 1

The aim of this exercise is to enable the participants to reflect on their own learning during the day.

Materials and setting

None required except a room large enough for all participants to sit in a circle so that they can see and hear each other clearly.

Method

Each person in turn is asked to complete the following statement and share it with the rest of the group: 'One thing which has happened to me during this day which has given me pleasure is . . .'.

Day 2 of the workshop would take place two weeks later. During the fortnight between the two days, suggested activities/homework were given as follows:

1   Participants were asked to read certain papers relating to the nursing process and care planning.
2   The participants were asked to be prepared to discuss on the next workshop day an incident or problem relating to the implementation of the nursing process which is either still unresolved or was resolved unsatisfactorily.
3   Each participant was asked to reflect on the following questions:
    How have I found the workshop so far?
    What is one thing I feel I have learned so far?
    Each participant was encouraged to keep a journal or diary on one facet of the nursing process which they were trying out in their unit between days 1 and 2 of the workshop.
4   Each participant was asked to write a care plan based on the nursing history they took on the afternoon of day 1 of the workshop.

Day 2

The second day of the workshop began with the following warm-up exercise.

WARM-UP EXERCISE

The aim of this exercise is to foster creative thinking, to help a group cohere prior to getting down to more serious work and to encourage participants to speak in the first person, e.g. 'I feel . . .' or 'I think . . .'.

Materials and setting

A room large enough for all participants to sit comfortably. The room should contain objects of everyday use or interest (pictures on the walls, a plant, desks, chairs, pens, books, briefcases, cups and saucers, and so forth). The exercise takes about 20 minutes, depending upon the size of the group.

Method

1   Each participant looks around the room and selects an object which interests her or catches her eye.
2   When everyone has chosen an object, each person takes it in turn to describe that object to the rest of the group. The description, however, must be in the first person, e.g. 'I am the plant sitting on the windowsill. I feel . . . when the sun shines on me and I feel . . . when I am watered regularly. My leaves are . . .' and so forth.
3   When each person has described an object in the first person, the participants should share with each other how they felt while doing the exercise. One way of doing this is for each person to complete the following statement out loud to the rest of the group:
'During this exercise I felt . . .'.

Following this warm-up exercise, the group spent some time feeding back their intersession work, after which ground rules were set for the rest of the day. The workshop facilitators introduced the idea of setting ground rules as a way of ensuring that everyone knew what to expect of the others and how to help the group function most successfully. The following ground rules were discussed and agreed:

- Each person speaks for herself and in the first person.
- Each person is responsible for making known her wants or learning needs and for negotiating these needs with others.
- Each person has the right to opt into or out of an activity.
- No personal information shared within the group is to be taken outside the group.
- All sessions commence and finish on time.

After coffee, the group continued to discuss some of the issues relating to change which they had begun to explore on the first day or had discovered during their intersession work. The brainstorming technique was used: this is a useful way of getting everyone's views or opinions about something in a non-threatening, non-judgemental way. The facilitator asks a question or for ideas about a topic and participants offer ideas as they come to mind. Each and every suggestion is written down on a large piece of paper or on the blackboard for all to see: all are written exactly as they are offered, in the same words used by the person making the response. All offerings are treated equally and are not judged or rejected in any way. For this particular brainstorming session, the following question was put to the participants who were asked to brainstorm ideas or answers:

Why do people find change difficult or uncomfortable and why do changes *not* take place in nursing?

Following this brainstorming session, the participants as a group discussed the ideas which arose from the brainstormed suggestions and sought clarification on some of the items from those who had offered them. The discussion ended with the drawing up of a list of factors which cause resistance to change.

The workshop then divided into small groups to carry out a planning-for-change exercise. Each group was asked to select from the list of factors causing resistance to change two reasons why people find change difficult. The groups then discussed how they might help to overcome these difficulties. From the discussion, each group drew up an action plan identifying the key strategies they might employ to prevent or manage resistance to change. A feedback session followed where each group shared their action plan and discussed their ideas about planning for change with the other groups. The session ended with a summary allowing the participants to take away a list of factors which cause resistance and suggested plans of action for overcoming such resistance.

The afternoon of day 2 began with a group ice-breaking exercise.

ICE-BREAKING EXERCISE

Called 'knots', the aim of the game is to encourage participants to work together to solve a problem.

Materials and setting

No materials are required. The room must be large enough to allow the group to stand in a circle.

Method

1   The participants stand in a circle facing inward. There must be an even number of people. If there are more than ten to twelve people, they should form into two groups to carry out the exercise; each smaller group, however, must have an even number of people.

2   Each person in the circle takes hold of the *right* hand of someone standing opposite to her in the circle with her own *right* hand.

3   Each person then takes hold of the *left* hand of a different person standing opposite to her with her *left* hand.

4   The task or problem of the group is to end up as a circle with people holding hands standing next to each other and with all hands and arms 'un-knotted'. Participants must not let go of anyone's hands in the process of un-knotting.

This was a lively exercise and was followed by the more serious problem-solving activity of the afternoon of day 2 of the workshop. The problem-solving activity was carried out in pairs. Each member of the pair identified one work problem related to introducing care planning and shared this problem with the other person in her pair. One of the pair spoke about her problem while the other listened without interrupting. When the first person finished speaking, the listener suggested ways of solving the problem. The pairs then reversed roles and the second person shared her work problem related to care planning. Examples of problems which were identified and shared were:

- Designing appropriate documentation for health visitors
- Coping with sisters who were actively resisting the use of care plans
- Motivating nursing auxiliaries to participate in discussions about care planning
- Helping nurses to evaluate their care

The afternoon ended with a summary of what had happened during the day and the opportunity for each participant to identify what she liked best and least about the day.

Intersession activities were suggested to prepare the participants for the third day of the workshop which was to take place two weeks later, including:

1   Continuing reading articles about the nursing process and care planning.
2   Specific articles and book chapters related to the management of change were also offered for further reading.
3   The participants were encouraged to select something they had learned during the workshop so far and were asked to try it out in their own work over the next two weeks.

Day 3

The third and final day of the workshop began with a reminder to the participants about the agreed ground rules, followed by a warm-up exercise:

WARM-UP EXERCISE

This is called the 'adverb' game, the aim of which is to have fun, get ready for more serious work and use one's imagination.

Materials and setting

None required except a room large enough for participants to sit in a circle.

Method

1   One person leaves the room. The other participants choose an adverb (a word which ends in 'ly', e.g. 'slowly').
2   The person returns and has to try to guess the adverb chosen by the rest of the group. She does

this by asking one person in the group 'What is your name?'.

3   The person asked gives her name but does it in a way suggested by the chosen adverb. She uses any manner, tone of voice or non-verbal gesture to give her name in a way which suggests the chosen adverb.

4   The person trying to guess can ask as many people in turn as she wishes until she has guessed the adverb.

The rest of the morning involved an exercise in pairs where each had the opportunity to practise 'selling' an idea to each other. The exercise involved one in the pair playing herself (as a nursing officer) and the other playing the part of a sister. The nursing officer had to 'sell' the idea of the Griffiths management restructuring of the NHS to the sister. The 'sister' was briefed to resist the idea. This exercise was carried out twice so that each participant could play both roles.

A feedback session followed which highlighted the difficulties in selling an idea to a 'reluctant' colleague, the problem of managing conflict and some of the very real and practical ways which can be employed to sell an idea.

The final session of the workshop was about leadership. It began with an activity in the form of a questionnaire which was designed to enable people to assess whether they are a task-orientated or person-orientated leader. The questionnaire is called a T-P (Task-Person) Questionnaire and can be found in Pfeiffer & Jones (1974). A brief discussion on leadership styles followed. The participants were then shown how to calculate their scores on the T-P Questionnaires. Further discussion followed, during which time the participants shared, if they so wished, their T-P scores and how they felt about the scores they had received and the implications of these scores for them. The discussion offered practical suggestions as to how they might go about changing their leadership orientation if they wished to do so.

The workshop ended with an opportunity for each participant to draw up her own action plan for her own work and development in terms of how she might better support her staff who are implementing care planning and how she might be better able to facilitate change.

Evaluation

The participants in the three-day workshop appeared to find it very useful. Comments included:

'Having advice on what to read both before and during the workshop was helpful.'
'It was extremely helpful to work with nursing officers from so many other specialities.'
'I found out a lot about myself.'
'I appreciated the value of the games, exercises and activities.'
'I got to know and trust people.'
'I enjoyed taking time out—not having a bleep for three days.'
'We did a lot of hard work together.'
'It's very rewarding working with these methods.'
'You could see people thinking and learning all the time.'
'Informal, friendly and safe environment.'

The workshop itself ended with each participant sharing one personal goal she had identifed for herself. This was followed by a 'goodbye' exercise:

GOODBYE EXERCISE

Each participant relates something nice or positive that she learned about someone else in the group. Ideally each participant should have something to say to every other participant.

Conclusion

Running a workshop in this way was a new experience for the facilitators and proved to be worthwhile for all concerned. The facilitators felt that certain activities were more successful than others but the greatest rewards came from sharing learning with the participants, watching them work together and learning to trust each other and to help each other solve problems of concern to them all. The workshop ended with enthusiastic and positive feelings of what they might be able to do in the future.

Nurse managers have learning needs and responsibilities with regard to care planning which are entirely different from those of clinical nurses. Nurse managers have to be given the opportunity to develop their own self-awareness and must be able to develop the skills required for leadership and for acting as agents of change. Using the experiential approach described in this chapter, nursing officers can develop such skills.

References

Pfieffer J & Jones J (1974) *A Handbook of Structured Exercises for Human Relations Training*, Vol I. San Diego: University Associates, pp. 7–12

Section V

Appendix

Role Play and De-roling

For many people, the idea of engaging in role play is fraught with horror and dread, both for the players, who cringe at the thought of performing in front of others, and for the teacher, who fantasises about 'opening cans of worms' about emotions which she may not be able to manage. Both of these are real fears born of inexperience in the appropriate use of role play.

The following are simple guidelines for successful, non-anxiety-provoking role play, designed to allow people to experience a situation in the relative safety of a classroom and then apply what they learn from the experience to their lives in the future.

1   Role play need not, and indeed should not, be carried out by a few people in front of a large audience. The most effective, non-threatening role play seems to be that which is performed by three or four people working together in privacy, with two or three playing parts in the situation and one or two acting as observers. No one else needs to watch.

2   Role play requires that the people involved trust each other and feel comfortable with each other. Therefore, the group needs time and experience working together so that they trust each other first. Many of the books and articles in the bibliography give suggested trust-building exercises for groups.

3   In any role play situation, the players must have

some sort of briefing about their role although they must be left free to play it as they wish. The observers must also have guidelines on how to be an effective observer. Chapter 9 offers guidelines for observers of role play.

4   Ground rules must be agreed beforehand, e.g. confidentiality about anything that happens in the role play. It is through the use of ground rules that people will feel safe in being honest in their role play.

5   Role play can be done by acting out a hypothetical situation or by using a real-life experience of one of the group. In the latter case, it is useful for the person who actually presents a real situation to play herself in the situation with other role players playing parts assigned to them by her.

6   Role play is only a useful learning experience if the individuals are given the opportunity to reflect on it, to discuss what happened for them and to draw up some plan of action for how they will in real life use what they have learned in the role play.

7   De-roling is essential after every role-play. De-roling is a way of ensuring that the feelings generated by playing a particular role are not taken away by the players after they have left the session, and that players can return—mentally and physically—to being themselves. De-roling takes place after the discussion. Thus the order of events is as follows:

(a)   Present the role play situation.
(b)   Select players and observers.
(c)   Brief players and give guidelines to observers.
(d)   Allow players a few minutes to think themselves into the role and get the feeling of the role.
(e)   Carry out the role play.
(f)   Allow players and observers time to discuss the role play and how they felt about it.
(g)   De-role players.
(h)   Action plan: how could we use what we learned from the role play in our future nursing?

De-roling techniques

There are many ways of enabling players to de-role and leave behind the roles they have played and the feelings which were aroused in the role play. A sample of de-roling techniques are offered here.

1   The most simple de-roling technique is for either the teacher or the observers of a role play to ask the following questions in turn of each person who has played a part:

'What is your name?'
Where are you?
What will you be doing this evening?

2   Another technique is for each of the players to write on a piece of paper all the feelings they were aware of in themselves during the role play. When everyone has done this, each person screws the piece of paper into a tight ball and throws it on the ground with force at the same time as shouting out her own name.

3   A third de-roling technique is similar to the second. Instead of writing their actual feelings on the paper, the role players write the following sentence:

'The feelings I had and saw demonstrated belong to role play.'

Each person then screws up the paper as described above and throws it on the floor with force at the same time shouting her name.

Conclusion

Role play is a powerful means of giving people the opportunity to come face to face with feelings and offers a practical way of trying out alternative ways of managing situations in the relative safety of a classroom. It requires trust and confidence on the part of students and teacher. Many teachers feel unable and afraid to use role play. The most appropriate way of developing the confidence to use role play, or any other experiential teaching method, is to experience these activities themselves as a member of a group. There are different ways by which teachers can do this. One way is for teachers to meet regularly with each other in small groups to try out role play and other experiential activities. If one or two teachers have already had experience of using these techniques, they can act as facilitators to the others. Once teachers have participated in role play themselves under skilled facilitation, they are in a better position to facilitate such sessions with their students. The same can be said for using any of the other exercises in this book. Once a teacher has participated in a role play she may become confident enough to practise leading such a session with a small group of fellow teachers as her practice group. The key seems to be in developing enough confidence to try methods such as this so that by doing it once or twice, confidence continues to grow.

A second useful resource is to explore courses which are available in a variety of places. Two such centres which offer courses to help teachers to become familiar with a variety of experiential methods, including role play, are:

Human Potential Research Project
Department of Educational Studies
University of Surrey
Guildford, Surrey

Contact person: Diana Lomax

ENB Learning Resources Unit
Chantrey House
798 Chesterfield Road
Sheffield S8 0SF

Contact person: Mrs M. Eastwood

Bibliography

This bibliography provides additional references and suggested reading related to all the issues raised in this book. The bibliography is divided into the following sections:

1   Interpersonal skills—general (including counselling and communication)
2   Self-awareness and personal growth
3   Stress management
4   Ethics and ethical decision-making
5   Humanistic psychology
6   Experiential learning
7   Nursing and education

For references specifically related to care planning and the nursing process the reader is referred to Hunt & Marks-Maran (1986) (see section on nursing and education below).

Interpersonal skills—general

Adler R, Rosenthal L & Towne N (1983) *Interplay*. New York: Holt, Rhinehart & Winston
Argyle M (1981) *Social Skills and Health*. London: Methuen
Argyle M & Trower P (1979) *Person to Person*. London: Harper & Row

Barnes D (1983) Teaching communication skills to student nurses. *Nurse Education Today*, **3** (2)

Bergman R (1977) Interpersonal relations in health care delivery. *International Nursing Review*, **24** (4)

Bridge W & Speight I (1981) Teaching the skills of communication, *Nursing Times* (Occasional Paper), **77** (32)

Burnard P (1985) *Learning Human Skills*. London: Heinemann

Cooper C (ed) (1981) *Improving Interpersonal Relations: Approaches for Social Skills Training*. Aldershot: Gower

Egan G (1976) *Interpersonal Living*. Monterey: Brooks Cole

Egan G (1977) *You and Me*. Monterey: Brooks Cole

Egan G (1986) *The Skilled Helper*. Monterey: Brooks/Cole

Eisler R & Frederiksen L (1980) *Perfecting Social Skills*. London: Plenum

Ellis R & Whittington D (1981) *A Guide to Social Skills Training*. London: Croom Helm

French P (1983) *Social Skills for Nursing Practice*. London: Croom Helm

Glaser S (1980) *Towards Communication Competency*. New York: Holt, Rinehart & Winston

Hargie O, Saunders C & Dickson D (1981) *Social Skills in Interpersonal Communication*. London: Croom Helm

Hays & Larsen K (1963) *Interacting with Patients*. New York: Macmillan

Jongward D & James M (1981) *Winning Ways in Health Care*. Menlo Park: Addison-Wesley

McLeod-Clark J (1981) Communication in nursing: analysing nurse-patient conversations. *Nursing Times*, **77** (1)

McLeod-Clark J & Bridge W (1981) *Communication in Nursing Care*. Chichester: John Wiley & Sons

Neeson B *et al.* (1984) Teaching communication skills to nurses. *Nurse Education Today*, **4** (2)

Porritt L (1984) *Communication: Choices for Nurses*. Melbourne: Churchill Livingstone

Rackham N, Honey P & Colbert M (1971) *Developing Interactive Skills*. Northampton: Wellens

Self-awareness and personal growth

Carkhuff R (1971) *The Development of Human Resources*. New York: Holt, Rinehart & Winston

Dickson A (1982) *A Woman in Your Own Right*. London: Quartet

Dye (1974) Self-concept, anxiety and group participation as affected by human relations training. *Nursing Research*, **23** (4)

Heron J (undated) *Life Styles Analysis*. Guildford: University of Surrey (Human Potential Research Project)

Heron J (1979) *Co-Counselling*. Guildford: University of Surrey (Human Potential Research Project)

Journard S (1971) *Self-Disclosure*. Chichester: John Wiley & Sons

Kalisch B (1971) Strategies for developing nurse empathy. *Nursing Outlook*, **19** (11)

Kilty J (1978) *Self and Peer Assessment*. Guildford: University of Surrey (Human Potential Research Project)

Layton J (1979) The use of modelling to teach empathy to nursing students, *Research in Nursing and Health*, 2

Scheirer M & Draut R (1979) Increasing educational achievement via self-concept change. *Review of Educational Research*, **49** (winter)

Turner S (1976) Fostering personal growth through small group interaction in a school of nursing. *Journal of Nursing Education*, **15** (6)

Wallston K *et al.* (1978) Increasing nurses' person-centredness. *Nursing Research*, **27** (3)

Stress management

Bailey R (1985) *Coping With Stress in Caring*. London: Macmillan

Bond M (1986) *Stress and Self-Awareness: A Guide for Nurses*. London: Heinemann

Cox T (1978) *Stress*. London: Macmillan

Ethics and ethical decision-making

Bergman R (1973) Ethics: concepts and practice, *International Nursing Review*, **20**, 5

Curtin L (1979) The nurse as an advocate. *Advances in Nursing Science*, **1** (3)

Curtin L & Flaherty M (1982) *Nursing Ethics: Theories and Pragmatics*. Bowie: Robert Brady

Fry S (1985) Individual vs. aggregate good: ethical tension in nursing practice. *International Journal of Nursing Studies*, **22** (4)

Hide E (1981) Teaching the ethical component of nursing. *Nurse Education Today*, **1** (3)

Rabb D (1976) Implications of moral and ethical issues for nurses. *Nursing Forum*, **15** (2)

Raths L (1966) *Values and Teaching*. New York: Merrill

Rumbold G (1986) *Ethics in Nursing Practice*. London: Baillière Tindall

Simons S, Howe L & Kirschenbaum H (1972) *Values Clarification: A Handbook of Practical Strategies for Teaching*. New York: Hart
Steele S & Harmon V (1983) *Values Clarification in Nursing*. New York: Appleton-Century-Crofts
Thompson I, Melia K & Boyd K (1983) *Nursing Ethics*. Edinburgh: Churchill Livingstone
Thompson J & Thompson H (1985) *Bioethical Decision-Making for Nurses*. Norwalk: Appleton-Century-Crofts
Uustal D (1978) Values clarification in nursing. *American Journal of Nursing*, **78** (12)

Humanistic psychology

Heron J (1985) *Six Category Intervention Analysis*. Guildford: University of Surrey, (Human Potential Research Project)
Rogers C (1961) *On Becoming a Person*. London: Constable

Experiential learning

Boud D (1973) *Experiential Techniques in Higher Education 1*. Guildford: University of Surrey (Human Potential Research Project)
Brandes D & Phillips H (1977) *Gamester's Handbook*. London: Hutchinson
Brandes D (1982) *Gamester's Handbook—II*. London: Hutchinson
Burnard P (1982) Through experience and from experience. *Nursing Mirror*, **156** (9)
Burnard P (1984) All that glistens. *Nursing Mirror*, **160** (20)
Connor M, Dexter G & Wash M (1984) *Listening & Responding*. York: College of Rippon and St John
Egan G (1985) *Exercises in Helping Skills*. Monterey: Brooks/Cole
French P (1980) A place for simulation in nursing education. *Nursing Focus*, **1** (11)
Gray J (1983) *Caring Communication*. London: DHSS (A teaching package for schools of nursing)
Heath J (1983) Gaming/simulation in nurse education. *Nurse Education Today*, **3** (4)
Heron J (1974) *Experiential Techniques in Higher Education II*. Guildford: University of Surrey, (Human Potential Research Project)
Heron J (1982) *Experiential Training Techniques*. Guildford: University of Surrey (Human Potential Research Project)
Hopson B & Scally M (1980) *Lifeskills Teaching Programme No. 1*. Leeds: Lifeskills Associates

Hopson B & Scally M (1980) *Lifeskills Teaching Programme No. 2.* Leeds: Lifeskills Associates

Kilty J (1982) *Experiential Learning.* Guildford: University of Surrey (Human Potential Research Project)

Pfeiffer J & Jones J (1974–1983) *A Handbook of Structured Experiences For Human Relations Training,* Vols I–IX. San Diego: University Associates

Satow A & Evans M (1983) *Working with Groups.* Manchester: Tacarde

Tomlinson A *et al.* (1984) Role play—learning to relate. *Nursing Times,* **80** (38)

Van Meuts M (1978) Role playing: playing a part as a mirror to meaning. *SAGSET Journal,* **8** (3)

Van Meuts M (1983) *The Effective Use of Role Play.* London: Kegan Paul

Nursing and education

Clark J (1975) *Time Out? A Study of Absenteeism among Nurses.* London: RCN

Gott M (1984) *Learning Nursing.* London: RCN

Hayward J (1975) *Information—a Prescription Against Pain.* London: RCN

Heath J (1982) Intention and practice in nursing education. *Nurse Education Today,* **2** (4)

Hunt J & Marks-Maran D (1986) *Nursing Care Plans: The Nursing Process at Work.* Chichester: John Wiley & Sons

Kershaw B & Salvage J (1986) *Models for Nursing.* Chichester: John Wiley & Sons

King V G & Gerwig N (1981) *Humanising Nursing Education.* Waterfield: Teacher's College Press

La Monica E (1985) *The Humanistic Nursing Process.* Boston: Jones & Bartlett

Orem D (1971) *Nursing: Concepts of Practice.* New York: McGraw Hill

Peplau H (1952) *Interpersonal Relationships in Nursing.* New York: Putnam

Redfern S (1981) *Hospital Sisters.* London: RCN

Roper N, Logan W & Tierney A (1985) *The Elements of Nursing.* Edinburgh: Churchill Livingstone

Index